D0211700

Laughing Your Way to Good Health!

by
Susan Vass

Table of Contents

About the Author . . .

Susan Vass is a woman who knows how to laugh at life. From behind a Sears electronic typewriter in her Minnesota home, she puts comic relief into even the most mundane daily events—the laundry, the kitchen, the kids. Public demand, however, often takes this talented author/comedienne out of the Midwest. Last year alone, she made over 75 personal appearances with such national acts as Robert Goulet, Andy Williams and the Smothers Brothers. Ms. Vass has performed for diversity of groups from schools and hospitals to Fortune 500 companies. For more information about the **Laughing Your Way to Good Health** program or to order additional copies of the book, contact Marketing Resources at (404) 457-6105 or write to us at 3301 Buckeye Rd., Ste. 202, Atlanta, GA 30341.

Published by
HMR Publications Group, Inc.

Illustrated by
Stephanie Allred

Copyright © 1989 Susan Vass
All Rights Reserved
4th Printing

Dedication and Acknowledgements

This may be my only book, the sum total of every humorous thought I have ever had in 42 years. I hope not. But, just in case, I want to dedicate this to some very special loved ones and to thank practically everyone who has ever made my stay on Planet Earth a little more pleasant.

TO: My mother, Dorothy Terry Baumbach, and my father, James, for giving me life and a sense of humor.

TO: Dorothy Saiko, for being my first non-professional standup role model; and to Phyllis Diller, Lily Tomlin, Minnie Pearl and the late Totie Fields for being my first professional female role models.

TO: My beautiful son, Jacob, for enriching my life immeasurably.

TO: My sister, Vicki Leigh Bloomquist, and her husband Lee; and my brother, James Terry Baumbach for constant love and support.

TO: Terri Vance, Kathy Haley and Jan Lok for believing in me.

TO: Bob Hansen and Clair Van Brocklin, the two best friends anyone could hope to have. The Ides of March and Halloween never produced two finer human beings. God Bless.

TO: Dave Barry, the world's funniest human.

TO: Colin and Nancy Covert for relentless nagging to "be all I can be."

TO: Leonard Cohen and Leo Kottke, for background music in my two most creative endeavors.

TO: Carol Scherfenberg, who has known me since we were 7, and loves me still.

TO: Haylie Cook, who makes order out of chaos, and who is my special little friend.

Laughing Your Way To Good Health:

The Introduction

If you have just bought this book, I thank you. If you are leafing through it trying to decide whether or not to spend the money, let me just promise you that you could not possibly invest in anything that would be more important. To me.

As for you, if it's a choice between this book or rent, food, clothes, etc., you probably better skip it. Of course, the amount of money you would spend on this book won't amount to squat toward rent and wouldn't even buy a decent meal at a fast food emporium, or make a dent in your truly-ridiculous credit card balance, so why not treat yourself?

As you page through this book, chuckling silently and then laughing right out loud, you should know that you are attracting the attention of the eagle-eyed sales personnel who right at this moment are worried that you are either about to walk off with it without paying or to require medical attention from hyperventilating during laughter. Why not just buy it and snort and cackle shamelessly in the privacy of your own home?

Some Questions You May Be Asking Yourself Right Now

Q: CAN I *REALLY* LAUGH MY WAY TO GOOD HEALTH?

A: I am not a doctor. If I were, I would be rich enough not to have to chain myself to an outmoded Sears electronic typewriter writing books. I make no medical claims whatsoever, but let's review what modern medicine does know about the mind-body connection.

For decades, *Reader's Digest* has been proclaiming that "Laughter is the Best Medicine," and it turns out that *Reader's Digest* may actually be right about something—isn't that amazing? (Remember, even a stopped watch is still right twice a day...)

In 1964, Mr. Norman Cousins, editor of *Saturday Review* became dreadfully ill with a disease of the collagen (that cottage cheese-like substance that holds our joints together). He was given a 1 in 500 chance of surviving at all, and was in great pain.

He felt that hospitals were pretty depressing places as a general rule (with the large exception of the one you are standing in, in the event that you are in a hospital gift shop thinking of buying this book...), and he subsequently checked himself out of the hospital and into a comfortable hotel.

With a partnership of his personal physician, his wonderful wife, and himself, he devised a personal recovery program which included massive doses of Vitamin C and nearly continuous bombardment of "humor therapy." He found that hearty laughter for 10 minutes afforded him two hours of pain-free sleep. He wrote an excellent book about his astonishing recovery called *Anatomy of an Illness* and then wrote a companion book called *The Healing Heart* about a similar recovery from a heart attack in 1979.

Subsequent research has shown many things about the benefits of frequent, hearty laughter. It appears that not only does a good belly laugh relax your whole body—inside and out—but it also burns 78 TIMES as many calories as you burn in a resting state. Mr. Cousins himself calls it "internal jogging."

There is also medical evidence that laughter produces more T-cells, an important part of the body's immune system. It may even stimulate the brain to produce endorphins which are the "natural drugs" which account for "runner's high." So: would you rather run a marathon and get all hot and sweaty—or laugh at this book for a few hours? The choice is yours.

Endorphins are sometimes referred to as the body's natural painkiller. Maybe years from now, dentists and surgeons will have patients watch "I Love Lucy" reruns or Eddie Murphy videos (depending on your taste) before extracting teeth and removing uteri.

After all, the French philosopher, Voltaire (known to his friends as a real kidder and "happening" guy), said, "The art of medicine consists of keeping the patient amused while Nature cures the disease."

Q: HEY, I'M SICK! HOW CAN YOU EXPECT ME TO LAUGH, YOU INSENSITIVE CLOD?

A: Good question. Say you have inadvertently had your nose removed ("Dr. Mel Pracktiss, that's rhino*plasty*, you nit, NOT RHINO*ECTOMY*"), when you came in to have it bobbed. First, get yourself a real good lawyer. Then, you might as well laugh at yourself, because everyone else is going to.

A: Even if you have a very serious disease—in fact, *particularly* if you have a very serious disease—what is to be *lost* by laughing? If it doesn't "work," will you have enriched or diminished your days by cheerfulness and laughter?

Q: WHAT IS THE CAPITAL OF MONTANA?

A: Helena.

Q: WHEN IS THIS BOOK GOING TO BE FUNNY?

A: Soon.

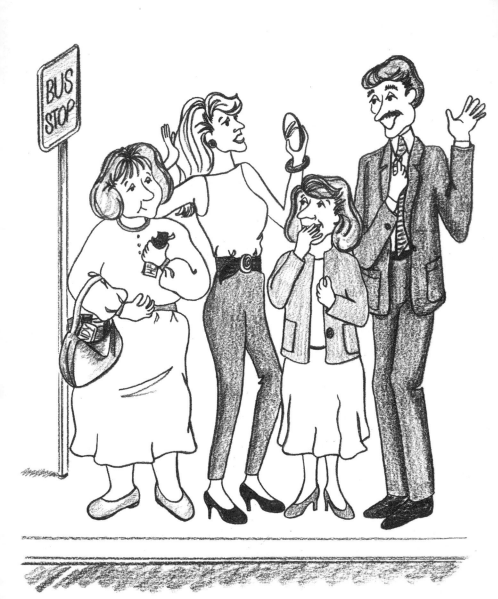

Chapter

1

Laughing Your Way Through Weight Loss And Gain

Make no mistake: achieving and maintaining a desirable weight is an enormous, daily, ongoing struggle.

The hefty among us are always looking for inspirational examples of people who have fought the good fight and won. Or lost, depending on your perspective.

I offer myself for your edification and inspiration. In 1988, I resolved to lose 30 pounds, and I'm thrilled to say that I only have to lose six more pounds. To get back to where I was when I made that promise.

Truth to tell, I have never met a woman who liked her own body. How about you, my friend? How about any of the people you know? Is there ONE woman who can look at herself naked in a full-length mirror and say, "I love my body. It's perfect!"?

The trouble is we don't think of ourselves as an integrated whole, but as a collection of parts, at least *some* of which are found wanting. If you are blessed with one of those cute, high round bottoms, then maybe your 32A chest is a source of endless angst. On the other hand, if you have a firm, perky bosom that hasn't migrated steadily south, then perhaps your thighs are a one-woman band when you wear corduroy. The point is, it's always something.

Let me give you some examples. One of my friends is 95 pounds. She's fit, she's trim, she works out every day. She has the kind of body I'd do ANYthing to have. (Except diet and exercise.) And she thinks she's too flat-chested.

Now, me I'm one of those "full-figured" gals who have helped give Jane Russell a second career hawking mega-bras. A lot of people think it would be pure heaven to be so full-figured. But I'm here to tell you that there are a lot of problems you may never have considered. For one thing, they don't make attractive lingerie for full-figured women.

This is just a fact. You go into the lingerie department, say, at Sears (maybe even nicer places than that), and you look at the stuff they have for the 32B's. Black lace. Silk. Satin. It's beautiful stuff! Your 42F's will go right through that stuff, just rip it all up. You go down to The House of Large Knockers, and the stuff they have in there is made out of sailcloth. Burlap. We're talking sturdy fabrics. And they have eight hooks. They're also full of hardware. Underwires, overwires, pulleys, winches. It's not a pretty sight.

And there's a lot of clothes you can't wear, too. Recently, I went shopping for Danskins® with one of my more modest-sized friends. Danskins®, you know, are those darling, shiny, leotard-like gar-

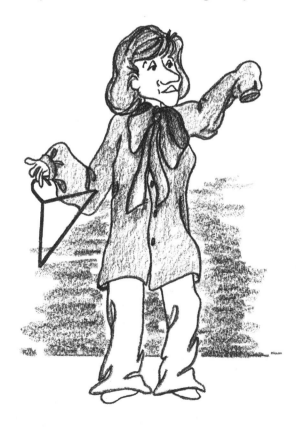

ments that look like they're painted on. They are made out of real tight material, so if you have any breasts at all, they start to panic because there's nowhere for them to go. One of mine went under my chin, and the other one around back.

I didn't get the outfit.

When you are voluptuous (as I call myself), or medically obese (as my doctor calls me), shopping for clothes can be a "Day in Hell." It is compounded if you are not only fat, but short as well. There are only three garments on earth made for the short and fat: the A-line (or, in some cases, A-frame) skirt, the muu-muu, and hospital gowns. Several of these garments are inappropriate in a corporate setting, the latter in particular, because it is invariably open in the back and comes only in Bile Green.

When you are short, hemming clothing becomes a second career. If, like me, you are 5'1" and your legs comprise only six of those inches—ankle-to-thigh—forget about buying chic, tapered or peg-legged pants. By the time you get them cut off and hemmed, the pant leg will be wide enough at the bottom for school-age children to play Hide-'N-Seek in.

Another hazard of being a Dachsund in a Greyhound fashion world is buying so-called fashion boots. I have a pair that went smartly up to the knees on the mannequin. On me, they're hip waders with stiletto heels.

So, I know what you're thinking. Buy Petites. Right? The Petites people are trying to be helpful, I know. They have scaled down the sleeves and inseams and all the detailing to a small, proportioned scale. The only problem here is that they also assume that Petites are teeny, tiny people without hips, breasts or thighs. Petites start in Size -2 and go all the way up to Size 4. Try getting a Petite Anne Klein silk jacket over a 42F chest. You look like an organ grinder's monkey.

I firmly believe that the Short *and* Fat clothes market is a market segment crying to be served by some clever entrepreneur. May I hasten the process by offering a few names for the new franchise: Massive Munchkins, Foxy Fireplugs, or simply, House of Large Petites.

Until that day, however, I plan to stick to hats, shoes, scarves, and jewelry on shopping binges. These are things which are not depressing to try on or to view in the neon glare of a merciless three-way mirror. I never met a scarf I didn't like. When I grow out of my scarves, THEN I'm going to go on a serious diet. When a 24-inch gold chain gets too tight around the neck, you'll find me either at a pricey health spa offering to sleep in a deck chair in exchange for a scholarship, or stapling my own stomach with my handy desk-top stapler.

It's no wonder we're all so neurotic about weight. What chance do we have to grow up with a healthy attitude toward it when the first thing that happens when we enter the world is that we're weighed? And then spanked.

They can't let you relax for five minutes! Welcome to the world baby, and get a fast start on skim milk and Gerber's Squash Lite.

A few months later, Mom will teach us a great baby game. She will ask us, "How big is my baby?" and we will learn to throw our arms above our heads as she says, "SO BIG!" Talk about mixed messages. Mom—the very center of our world—is absolutely ecstatic that we are BIG. If we fail to scarf up one bite of our strained beets, she will pretend our spoon is an airplane or a dump truck and force open our little mouths. She will persist in feeding us the very same bite of beets several times, if necessary, despite body language (repeatedly spitting it out) that would be clear even to a person of the most limited intelligence.

Surely you will agree with me that this weight problem is not my fault! Besides the previous discussion about simply being too short for my weight, I should point out that I also have a large frame. I know that I have a large frame because whenever I find my weight on those charts, I read over and it says, "large frame."

I am also married and that's very fattening. I gained 25 pounds. At the reception. It was kind of a surprise to my husband, too, of course.

Moreover, I had a baby recently, and gained a whopping 45 pounds during pregnancy. Okay, not that recently—he's in 10th grade now. But I believe that weight lost slowly will stay off better.

I know there is a group of lifelong dieters out there who can identify with everything I am saying. Sadly, there is also a much smaller group, shaking their heads and pursing their tight little lips—lips that have NEVER been the first stop for a whole bag of Mallomars. The group I refer to is The Naturally Thin.

I think you know who you are. And, there's something I think you should know about yourselves. People hate you. There. I've said it. And I'm not sorry. Because frequently, The Naturally Thin have a very superior attitude. For example, the scrawny little carry-out boy at my supermarket last week. He looked at my eight bags of groceries, and asked, "Would you like to drive up for these, Ma'am, or were you planning on eating them right here?"

See what I mean? That's exactly the kind of attitude *I* can do without. You also get a lot of bad advice from The Naturally Thin. My hairdresser, Karin, is a beautiful woman, almost six feet tall, thin, blonde, gorgeous.

"Karin," I begged, "Tell me your secret: HOW do you stay so thin?"

And this is the valuable advice she gave me.

"Well, Susan, sometimes I just get so busy I forget to eat."

Get real! NEVER once, in 42 years, have I forgotten to eat. Although I have, on occasion, forgotten that I've already eaten. That's why I never really learned to swim. My mother always made me wait an hour after eating.

I blame some weight gain on those catchy Armed Forces commercials that exhort you to "Be All You Can Be," although my naturally thin friends point out that doesn't necessarily mean "Be As Big As You Can Be."

Being overweight can sometimes lead you to be less than honest. I live in mortal terror that one day I will be pulled over for some minor traffic infraction and the policeman will scream, "What have you done with Susan Vass? It says on her license she weighs 105, so *YOU* CAN'T BE SUSAN VASS!" It's so easy to make a clerical error on your application form. 150—105—so, I'm selectively dyslexic.

Suffice it to say that I'm never going to be asked to be in one of those ads that say, "Don't Hate Me Because I'm Beautiful." Is that obnoxious, or what?! Those models should be confined and force-fed pork rinds and whipped cream until you can't see their collar bones any more.

Which reminds me of the latest therapy group I read about. Get this: it's a support group for people who are "too attractive!" Now there's an oppressed minority you can really feel sorry for. Immediately I wondered how you get in. Do the other too attractive people have to vote on you? Or, if *I* believe that being too attractive is a major problem for *me*, is that good enough?

The article went on to complain that the too attractive are discriminated against in employment. This could open up a whole new market for plastic surgeons and orthodontists to treat people who want to have big hook noses and/or buck teeth. Then they can just watch those job offers come rolling in!

My advice to the too attractive who want to graduate from their support group real fast is to follow me around for a month and eat everything I eat. I guarantee that within four short weeks the only

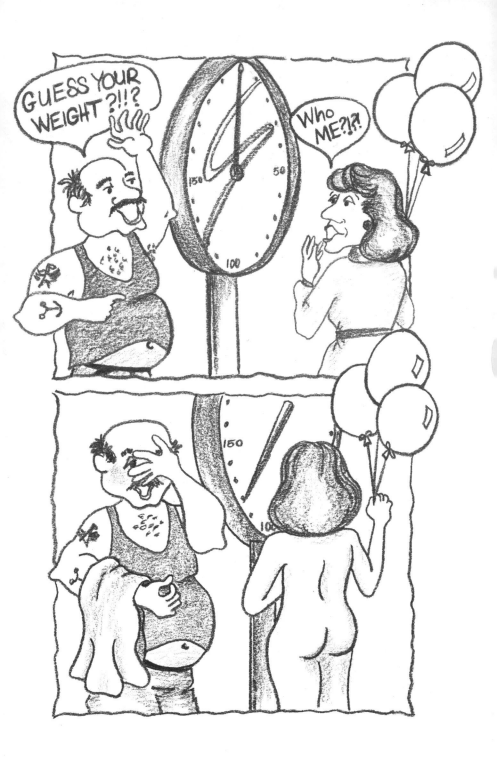

"support" you will need is from an 18-hour, long-line bra.

The group is also sponsoring a lecture by Erik Estrada on "How Unfair It Is That People Think the Incredibly Attractive are Dumb." That lecture will begin when the big hand is on the 12 and the little hand is on the 8.

You do have those moments in your life when you know you really have to do something about your weight. I had such a day of reckoning at our Minnesota State Fair. I was having a terrific time, eating my way down the Midway, when from nowhere this sleazebag with tattoos everywhere, including his nose, calls out to me, "Guess your weight, madame?"

"Well," I replied curtly, "If you guess that number outloud, you can also jolly well try to guess how many minutes you have left to live."

Then I wandered around the fairgrounds appreciating the butter sculpture of Princess Kay of the Milky Way, the fragrantly scented live animal barns, the Cotton Candy, Pronto Pups, Mini-Donuts, Caramel Apples, and one more Corn Dog for the road. Finally, I passed the scruffy weight-guesser again and I felt sorry for him because he didn't seem to be getting any business and clearly he needed the money to pay for another tattoo, like, on his tongue.

So, I said, "Okay, give it your best shot. What do you think I weigh?"

And you know what? He guessed four or five pounds HIGH! I was pretty darn excited what with winning that festive plastic beer mug on the line and all.

Of course, to be fair to the fellow, I don't think he expected that I would weigh NUDE. It was quite a surprise to him, and to the other fairgoers.

I think, if we're honest, we pretty much all weigh naked, don't we? Completely nude, first thing in the morning, before we put on our deodorant, and after we've gone to the bathroom. Sometimes I even weigh before *and* after. Just to record any little loss. Something like that can just make your whole day.

Anyway, I came to a point where I needed a support group.

So, I joined TOPS. Not the one that stands for "Take Off Pounds Sensibly." No, this is kind of a less well-known chapter of that— "Tomorrow Or Pretty Soon." The nice thing about this particular TOPS is that because we're always starting "tomorrow", *every* day is "the day before you start a diet", in which you feel perfectly justified in consuming everything in sight without guilt since any minute now you are going to be severely deprived.

This TOPS group is just my speed, which is to say: gradual. I plan to lose a pound every solar eclipse. We are also working on a gradual exercise program using Shelley Winters' new book *Thin Thighs in 30 Years*. You do one leg lift every other day or walk briskly to your mailbox and back. Remember: be careful not to work up a sweat, therefore you need not launder your clothes as often.

The TOPS group gives you a calorie counter. Scientists have computed the exact number of calories in every food known to Man. For example, they have figured out the number of calories in *one* chocolate chip cookie. It is of no concern to me how many calories there are in *one* chocolate chip cookie. What I need to know: how many calories are there in a *batch* of chocolate chip cookies? And, are there fewer in the dough?

But the silliest calorie count I ever saw was on a Hershey Bar. I was having my morning Hershey, when I happened to glance at the nutrition panel to see if I was actually fulfilling my minimum daily requirement for something like riboflavin, and there was the calorie count: 140 calories *in a serving*. And right below that, it boldly stated: two servings! Sure. Like, I'm going to eat *half*, and save the rest for another day. Like I could sleep knowing it was there.

If you closely examine your candy bar you will also notice in tiny print the opportunity to return the unused portion of your candy bar if, for some reason, it is unsatisfactory to you, and guess what they'll do? Send you another one! Isn't that a great example of logic at work in our daily lives?

"I don't like this; what I really want is MORE."

So, I ate it all except for a tiny corner and sent that in with a letter assuring them that I had given it a *really* good try, but upon examining my true feelings, found that I had not been satisfied after all. With an initial investment of only 40¢ and a series of post office boxes, you can keep one Hershey Bar going for the rest of your life.

Awhile back I mentioned riboflavin, just to prove I could spell it, and to make me appear hip to the whole subject of nutrition. I have never seen either a "riboflavin" or Yugoslavia, but reliable sources inform me that both exist. I suspect that when other vitamins were being discovered by Madame Curie or Eli Whitney that the Riboflavin Council got together to lobby the folks who were inventing the minimum daily requirement and pointed out that it would be in everyone's best interest if they included riboflavin.

Then they could make up a list of foods allegedly containing riboflavin and convince health food writers that if consumers didn't rush right out and ingest thousands of milligrams of riboflavin weekly, they would get narcolepsy or their private parts would atrophy. So pretty soon people would flock to health food stores in a frantic search for riboflavin in much the same way they are stockpiling oat bran.

Lately, I have been very concerned about this calcium deficiency thing—osteoporosis. So, I try to eat about a gallon and a half of Haagen Dazs a day. Just for the calcium. In fact, if it's Rum Raisin, you'll get your iron there too.

Ice cream is my great downfall on any kind of weight loss program. Have you ever taken one of those long-handled iced tea spoons and gone *mining* for the fudge in the Fudge Ripple? I like to eat all the fudge in a kind of surgical strike, squish it down, and then tell the family it was Vanilla.

Here's another diet tip: if you are on one of those really low-calorie diets, try to have 50 or 60 chocolate chip cookies a day. This keeps up your spirits and prevents you from going on a diet-busting *binge.*

I find I am able to stay on a diet pretty well during the day. It's that night eating that really trips me up. I get home late from a book-signing or performance; my family is asleep; and I go *foraging* for food, like a small forest animal. How many others of you have ever eaten sweetened condensed milk right out of the can? It makes a fine snack in a real emergency when you don't have the butter, sugar and graham cracker crumbs necessary to actually make one of the recipes on the can.

My main problem is that I am a binge eater. I have semi-bulimia. I just do the binging part. The worst binge I ever went on in my life started when my husband invited ten people from his law office over for dinner. Now, even though I love to eat, I am not that good a cook. In fact, when my son was very small, whenever I would go *near* the stove, he'd say, "Hot, hot!"

However, desserts are my best thing, culinarily-speaking. So, I did my best with the dinner and then made my specialty for dessert—chocolate cheesecake. This is a really special cheesecake. It has 40 ounces of cream cheese. You can actually watch people get bigger while they're eating it. It has cream in every form known to man—cream cheese, sour cream, and whipped cream on top. It is so rich that the 12 of us only ate half of it.

The next day, my husband went to work and I was alone with the cheesecake. So, I had a little piece for breakfast—who wouldn't? Then I had another little mid-morning snack—about 7:30 a.m. At that point, it was all *raggedy,* so I had to even it up. I mean, we can't have that unsightly mess now, can we? What if "House Beautiful" came by and saw a raggedy cheesecake? There goes the two-page color spread.

Then I ate a piece standing up—that doesn't count. Pretty soon, to my horror and disbelief, I had eaten all the cheesecake. My husband would be coming home soon, and this is not the kind of item that is burglarized from your home.

I thought of trying, "Oh, honey, it was awful—they tied me up and everything..."

But, he's a pretty smart guy, and I didn't think he'd buy that. So what did I do? I BAKED ANOTHER ONE AND ATE IT DOWN TO HALF!

Even non-binge eaters find it difficult to get well-balanced meals on the road—unless you count "balance" as a Twinkie in one hand and a Ho-Ho in the other. Here's a tip for frequent travelers: never eat in any restaurant called "Mom's." If you don't eat all your lima beans, they don't let you order dessert.

My favorite dessert, next to ice cream, is pie. Preferably pie with ice cream so I don't have to agonize over my decision between them. I wouldn't want to say I spend a lot of time at Baker's Square, our local pie shop, but last week I paid off my electric bill in returned pie tins.

It was a large bill, too, because our whole house is a salute to electricity. My motto is "It is better to leave *all* the lights on than to curse the darkness." Each light bulb is a tiny eternal flame in memory of all the money we *could* have had.

I don't know about your area of the country, but in Minnesota, the power company gets a rate hike approximately every fifteen or twenty minutes. Then they use this money to put out helpful brochures with great ideas for cutting down on your electric bill, such as "Don't run your air conditioner in the summer." Why didn't I think of that? Or, "Turn off appliances when not in use." But, if you're like me, before you go to work in the morning, you like to get out the iron, the mixer, and the blender and leave them running all day.

Back to the subject of dieting. Let's say you have really, really decided this time to lose some weight. How to start? Well, here's some cheery news from medical science: DIETS DO NOT WORK. Here's why:

Nature. Yup, it's just that simple. Dieting is completely unnatural and your body knows this and will not put up with it.

Every body has a rate at which it burns fuel which is called its "metabolism." Some lucky people have very high metabolisms and burn fuel really inefficiently, like a big, drafty house with the thermostat set to 85 degrees and no weatherstripping or caulk. No matter how much "fuel" in the form of pasta, chocolate and french fries are stoked into someone with a high metabolism, they can't seem to store any extra "fuel" in the form of fat. (Think here of your own savings account—no matter how much you put in, somehow it gets all used up.)

If we were to have a serious famine, these people with high metabolisms would be dead within minutes.

My body, on the other hand, is like a big Volkswagen. It uses so little fuel that it could go cross-country on one tank of gas. So, it makes my hips and thighs into extra fuel tanks. I am the kind of person who could be discovered alive several months after an earthquake.

"We are just flabberghasted," the rescue workers would say, "Ms. Vass only had three Wheat Thins and a Salted Nut Roll, and not only did she live for five months trapped in this basement, but she only lost four pounds. She could use a bath, though..."

Women particularly are blessed by Nature with low metabolic rates. It seems that women need a certain percentage of body fat (apparently around 75%) in order to sustain the wonderful female processes which guarantee the continuation of the species—ovulation, menstruation, PMS, things like that.

Long, long ago when Nature just got started, the human race was a very fragile group what with getting nearly wiped out with nauseating frequency by floods, famine, pestilence, and rabid dinosaurs. When primitive cavepersons didn't know how to grow stable food sources, like pizza, they relied too heavily on being able to find, track and kill large, ugly animals. So, in order that women didn't starve between successful hunts, Nature decreed that women should have this extra fat to use as fuel. Because, God forbid women should cease having the joy of periods while they were starving.

Nature is a very slow learner. Nowadays, when a woman stops eating for a few days, in order to burn her already-stored fuel, Nature right away gets alarmed and thinks, "Famine!" And can you guess what Mr. Metabolism does then? He *slows down,* because he is afraid that it will be a very long time until this woman gets to eat again. So, pretty soon, instead of living on a modest 56,000 calories a day, as the woman was accustomed to doing, the body is now training itself to live on 1500 calories a day—*without burning any stored fat.*

Wait, it only gets worse!

Pretty soon this woman gets tired of having the energy level of a slug on Quaaludes, gets sick to death of eating cucumber slices dipped in plain yogurt, and reverts back to her normal eating pattern of six large meals and 23 snacks a day. If she has managed to lose any weight at all, while cutting her calories down to 1500, she now gains it all back in 15 minutes, because she has now trained her body to do just fine on 1500 calories so anything over that will be stored as—you guessed it—fat. Next time, she will have to cut down to 700 calories, then 200 calories, and so on. You get the depressing picture.

Moreover, Nature is so protective of women's layer of fat that when a woman cuts down to starvation levels, the body will devour anything handy to avoid dipping into the fat—things you may have a use for later like the pancreas and biceps. It will eat up muscle tissue just like a Pac-Man and then when you go back to regular eating, do you think it will replace that muscle tissue? No can do. It will replace it all right—with fat. That is why diets don't work. Every "diet" actually and truly makes you fatter! If you diet long enough, you will be a walking, talking, bouncing bag of blubber.

Doctors know this; but they don't have a better idea. So, when you consult them about being overweight, they will put you on a diet, knowing full well that you will fail. This is why all the diet pills, powders, books, and clinics are a mega-buck "growth" industry.

So, before you fall into the diet trap once again, ask yourself if it's really time to go on a diet. Here are some handy clues:

YOU KNOW IT'S TIME TO GO ON A DIET WHEN...

- You take off all your clothes, and you still feel dressed.

- Children ask you to jump in the pool. So they can bodysurf.

- People stop asking you to "pull your own weight" in a project, because they think that would be an unfair share.

- The "inch" you can pinch is on your elbow.

- You have more chins than children.

- You outgrow your socks.

WHEN IS A GOOD TIME TO BEGIN A DIET?

- If it's Tuesday or later in the week, a good time to begin is next

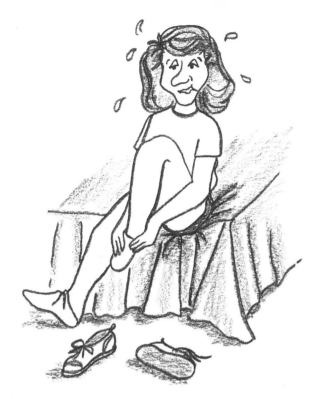

Monday.

- If it's the 17th of the month or later, a good time to begin is the first of next month.

- If it's any month between August and December, a good time to begin is the first of next year.

- If it's within three to ten weeks of a major holiday such as Christmas, Mother's Day, or National Pork Bellies Day, a good time to begin is after the holidays.

- If you have a major class reunion coming up, a good time to begin is last week. (Remember: you do not *have* to go to class reunions. How many of those geeks did you really *like*, anyway?)

- January is one of the most popular months to begin a diet. It's after the holidays, the first month in a brand, spanking new year, the year in which you finally lose weight, write that Great American Novel, organize your closets and quit smoking. You know it's January when your shopping cart has $300 worth of Lean Cuisine and 14 bags of Mallomars, for (wink, wink) the kids.

HOW DO I PICK A DIET?

This is very difficult what with the Macrobiotic Diet, the Beer and Chip Diet, the Low Carbohydrate/High Protein Diet, the High Carbohydrate/Low Protein Diet, the Fig Newton/Watercress Diet, the Isaac Newton Apple Diet, the Newton Minnow "bad TV" Diet, and Anorexia, to name just a few. Let's examine several of the major contenders:

THE WATER DIET: *All* diets say "Drink 8 to 10 glasses of water a day." This is to give you the illusion of fullness, to give you something to do with your mouth periodically, in lieu of stuffing it, and, as a side benefit, to fill up your ankles. The Water Diet just takes that concept to its logical extreme. You must drink 8 to 10 *quarts* of water a day. This one works best if you are not planning to be away from your bathroom for over 15 minutes at a stretch.

THE SCARSDALE DIET: This one just sounds so upscale you know it has to work. Think of all those chic people who can't be "too rich or too thin." They must know what they're doing, right? The diet just wouldn't have the same panache if it were the Cleveland Diet or the Minneapolis Diet.

Minneapolis correctly conjures up images of sturdy, blonde Scandinavians eating bland, yet caloric food. A Minnesotan is not troubled by boring cuisine. In fact, a meal of plain boiled potatoes, boiled cauliflower, boiled cod in white sauce and tapioca pudding with whipped nondairy topping is considered close to ideal as its color best approximates the frozen landscape we enjoy for seven months of the year. A sprig of parsley tossed whimsically upon this sea of white is considered entirely too festive, although among some Lutheran sects it is thought to be a lucky foreshadowing of Spring.

It is not true that the Scarsdale Diet entails shooting your unfaithful lover and then losing weight by eating prison food.

DR. ATKINS' DIET REVOLUTION: This is a diet, which, on the surface, does seem like a "revolution" because you can eat all the protein and fat you want! Butter, eggs, cheese, steak—even whipped cream! But no fruits, vegetables or carbohydrates. After every previous diet of unlimited celery, kiwi, and Bibb lettuce, this one has great appeal until you realize that the very foods that are prohibited are the ones you would kill for. On this diet, it won't matter how long you are away from your bathroom, because *nothing* is going to be happening in that department, if you get my drift. There is absolutely no roughage in either steak or cheese and very soon you will need small-scale explosives to get anything moving through your nether regions.

Furthermore, your cholesterol will shortly be in five digits, like your Zip Code. You will have to take a really hot bath just to melt your blood enough to get it moving in the morning.

WEIGHT WATCHERS: This is an excellent, time-tested program which allows a wide variety of foods with the calories reduced by a sensible amount, combined with group cheerleading. This is all led by an "instructor" who used to be fat, but now is merely underpaid for conducting the support sessions.

Unfortunately, the Weight Watchers in MY neighborhood is held at the Moose Lodge. You drive up and the sign says "Moose Parking." No way, José. I don't need this aggravation.

Wouldn't it be loverly if we could go on One Final Diet and then never be fat again no matter what we ate? Sadly, it never works that way. Noooooo...the fat always come back—Desperately Seeking Susan.

You know you're on a strict diet when "toothpaste" is listed as a "snack."

Whenever I'm on a real low-calorie regimen, I dream about food. Once, I dreamed I was at an all-you-can-eat buffet. I had my plate heaped with forbidden comfort foods like meat loaf and mashed potatoes and gravy, cherry Jello with bananas and marshmallows, and a big slice of lemon meringue pie, when an employee snatched my plate away!

"Hey," I cried, "I thought this was all-you-can-eat."

"It is," he said, "And that's all you can eat."

Lucky thing, too, because as it was, when I woke up I had gained three pounds.

I have also heard of a new Garlic and Bleu Cheese Diet. You don't lose any weight, but you look a lot smaller from a distance.

The human mind is a wonderful tool which can rationalize anything. When you're on a rigid diet that prohibits desserts, it's this ability to rationalize which enables you to count a caramel pecan roll as a "bread." And a Snicker as a "vegetable"—because of the peanuts. Sure, peanuts are a very important member of the "legume" family.

On a diet, weighing in too often is discouraged. Most diet professionals recommend weighing no more than once a week. The reason for this is if you weigh more than you think you should after suffering for several days you think, "Phooey (or words to that effect), no matter how disciplined I am, it is useless. I may as well go have that Hot Fudge Sundae." On the other hand, if that scale comes to rest on a number *lower* than the one you were dreading, you think "Boy, I'm way ahead of my scheduled weight loss. I think I will treat myself with a tiny hot fudge sundae."

I try to limit weighing in to no more frequently than say, commercial breaks in a Super Bowl.

Some diet experts recommend journaling as a way of charting your progress and recording your feelings during the ordeal.

Here are my actual monthly entries from my last (as in, "most recent," not "final") diet:

June 8th— It is hot today. I *must* lose 27 pounds. I feel optimistic that this time I will make it.

July 8th— Very hot and humid today. Perhaps it might be more pleasant if we took off the storm windows. I must lose 35 pounds.

Aug. 8th— I must lose 42 pounds. By Sunday.

For some reason, whenever I start a big diet, I get a cold. Then, I'm really in a quandary. I never know whether it's "Feed a cold, starve a fever," or the other way around. So I just feed 'em both. You don't want to take a chance on making a mistake when it comes to your health. In fact, when I have a cold, a fever and a sore throat, I figure I should be eating for four.

The diet experts all say "eat *only* when you're hungry," which I equate with making love only when you want to have a baby. What has hunger got to do with eating, anyway? Eating is a pleasurable activity. I love to eat. I live to eat. I don't understand people for whom that's not the case. For example, those jerks in the TV commercial where they're holding their heads, frowning, trying to decide, "Stuffing or potatoes? Stuffing or potatoes?" Have them both, for God's sake! Put gravy over the whole works!

Another annoying group of people? Cookbook writers. They feature a recipe for a teeny, tiny casserole and say "Serves six to eight." Six to eight WHAT? Anorexic midgets, maybe. Or one teenage boy.

We have now spent considerable time discussing the problem of being overweight. Popular slogans notwithstanding, I believe that it is possible to be "too thin," just as George Steinbrenner and Imelda Marcos are obviously living refutations of the notion that you cannot be "too rich."

So, how do you know if you're too thin, instead of just fashionably emaciated?

Here are a few good clues:

YOU ARE TOO THIN WHEN:

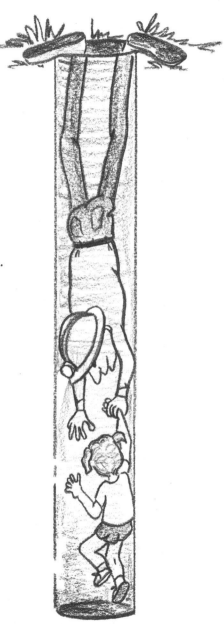

- Diana Ross looks like a real porker standing next to you.
- Barbie's Malibu maillot fits you.
- You could have gone down the drainpipe to rescue Baby Jessica.
- Your legal limit of alcohol is 1 teaspoon of a wine spritzer.
- Your promising career as a concert pianist is cut short because your fingers get stuck in the space *between* the keys.
- You can wear a charm bracelet. As a belt.
- Your only concept of the word "bust" is when Don Johnson breaks down the door to the home of a Miami cocaine dealer.
- You describe Olive Oyl as "full-figured."
- Panhandlers give *you* money and tell you to get a hot meal.
- You can set a snack tray on your collarbone.

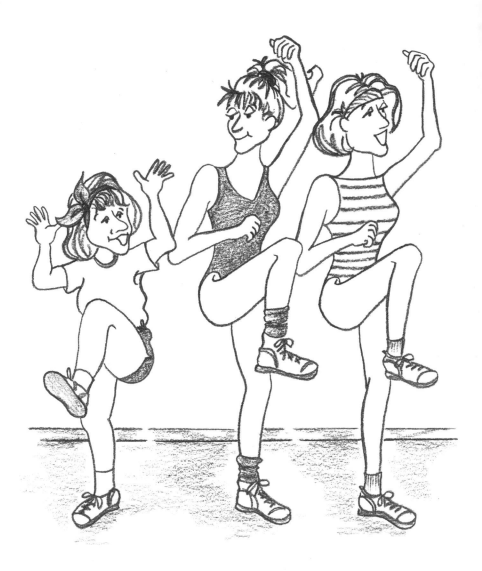

Chapter
2

Laughing Your Way Through Exercise

As we finish out the '80's and head into the '90's, it is no longer enough just to be skinny. Now, you have to be fit as well—something I consider to be just one more enormous burden. At first, I thought fitness was just a fad, and I thought I'd sit it out in much the same way I have decided to take a pass on the reintroduction of the mini-skirt. But, it's been about 15 years now and fitness seems to be more of a trend than a fad, so I figure it's time to get with the program.

As luck would have it, I am married to a fitness fanatic. He runs five miles a day, every day, even in Minnesota in the winter (September-July). When a male person runs in 60 below zero wind chill, he runs a serious risk of extreme personal injury in an unusually sensitive region. My runner has fashioned an attractive "mitten" for that region out of an old pair of earmuffs, so he no longer faces the kind of painful frostbite Adam might have endured if the Garden of Eden had been in Anchorage.

My husband is such a fitness fanatic that he's even into sports nutrition. He has this new book *Eat to Win* authored by someone who claims to have trained every major athlete since Atlas. "Eating to win" does not appeal to me. Frankly, I am just not that competitive. "Eat to place," "eat to show" is good enough for me.

Joggers are the absolute worst for snotty attitudes. Catch the looks they give you when you're driving. Looks that seem to say,

"This would be a great road if it weren't for the CARS on it."

I run five feet a day because I think you should be able to run the length of your own body. Like most of us, even though I don't exercise much, I do buy a lot of exercise books. It counts, doggone it! I had this urge to exercise just the other day. I said, "I need a new exercise book!" So, I got in the car, drove three blocks, and looked over the selection at my favorite bookstore. I only had $45, so I knew I could only get one. I was trying to decide between Arnold Schwarzenegger's *Body Building for Women* and *Thin Thighs in 30 Days*. I finally chose the body building one. I figured then if anyone mentioned my thighs, I could beat the crap out of them.

The kind of exercise books that really bug me are celebrity beauty books where some naturally gorgeous woman like Raquel Welch or Linda Evans tries to tell the rest of us mere mortals how to look great by following her routine. I could do Raquel's yoga workout for 23 hours out of every 24 and there is no way I am going to come close to looking like her without major surgery in numerous areas. For openers, her *arms* are longer than my *legs*.

All the exercise in the world cannot produce prominent cheekbones or long legs. So, resist the temptation to compare yourself with God's Gifts. Besides, have you *seen* Jane's and Raquel's (now-ex) husbands? Hey, I'm no Ms. America myself, but I must point out that chances are excellent that *your* man—even in his undershirt—is better-looking than theirs!

I want to see a celebrity beauty book by someone who starts out looking like Ma Kettle and by religiously following the program, ends *up* looking like Raquel. Now *that* I'd buy.

It is my intention to get in shape very soon now, before I acquire an unfortunate nickname like William "The Refrigerator" Perry. A moniker like that is all well and good for a football player, but I do not care to be named after a major appliance. Luckily, I am too short to ever be called a refrigerator. I would probably be called Susan "The Dryer" Vass. Something short and squat with a tendency to overheat.

I saw a poster advertising a local workout salon with a real macho dude flexing his muscles and the caption read, "I sweat for this body!" Big deal. I sweat going up a flight of stairs. The only other time I sweat is when I start to panic about missing a meal.

I finally decided to join an exercise club. I picked the one Cher does the ads for. We're often mistaken for each other at the club:

"Gee, is that Susan Vass or Cher?" people cry, "We can't tell."

It's a very exclusive, expensive club. It costs $250 a session.

Okay, it costs $500 a year and I've only used it twice. The exorbitant sign-up fee is part of the weight-loss strategy. It costs so much to join that you can't afford food.

I try to spend an hour at the club every day now. That includes a 10-minute whirlpool, 10-minute sauna, and 40 minutes circling the parking lot looking for a space near the door.

The club is filled with enough torture devices to make a South American dictator's heart beat wildly with joy and anticipation. I guess it *is* time for Nautilus though when you slap a mosquito and only wound it.

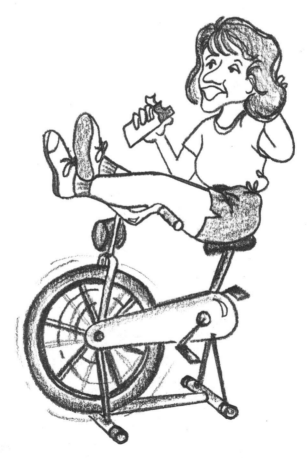

Then there are the exercise bikes. My club has many varieties, but my favorite is the digital, state-of-the-art model where you can program it for varying degrees of difficulty. I put it on the "downhill" mode; put my feet up on the handlebars; and have a couple of Snickers for the trip. It's important to keep your strength up during an activity like that.

I do enjoy the swimming pool. I usually stay in the special "floaters" lane, trying not to run my air mattress into the irritable lap swimmers who invariably splash water on my sandwich when they do their show-off kick turns.

According to fitness gurus, walking is supposed to be as good for you as running, and less stressful on your joints. However, in order to "walk off" the calories in my average lunch, I'm supposed to walk to Milwaukee. And back.

I grew up in a small town where nobody ever walks *anywhere.* If you were invited more than two doors down for dinner—you piled everybody in the car and drove. We didn't get "tennis elbow" or "football knees," but we did occasionally slam our fingers in the car door.

The latest exercise craze to overtake the country is aerobics, an activity based on the premise that hopping and flailing around to badly-recorded disco music burns more calories than sitting still. The adventure begins the first moment you examine your thighs as they squoosh out the French-cut legholes of your little leotard like toothpaste out of a tube. It is dismaying to discover that your cellulite has cellulite. This is a sight which should inspire you to a really vigorous workout, however, the effect on me is to head speedily for the exits. This feeling is further enhanced by an apparent state law in Minnesota (I can't speak for your particular state) that reads "all aerobics instructors have to be tan, gorgeous 19-year-old blonde Nazis." They make you do things which are prohibited by the Geneva Convention.

For example, after making you do 10,000 situps, the instructor actually has the nerve to ask, "How many people want *more* abdominal work?" And every time, some scrawny Yuppie bitch squeals, "Yes, yes, we want more!" I recognized her too—she's the one who about a minute before the bell rang would say, "Sister Colma, you forgot to give homework." (Do you remember her now?)

You look around at the other women in the class and wonder, "Where did all these young, thin women come from? And why don't they go back there?" Are they really members or does the club just rent them? Maybe they travel from club to club making the rest of us feel like big, old 78 rpm records amidst all the 45's on the Turntable of Life.

And their outfits! There's not enough spandex in those leotards for a decent Barbie outfit. Any second you expect a voice to come over the PA system and say, "Will the short, dumpy lady in the pink sweatsuit please get behind a pillar? For heaven's sake, we're conducting a prospective members tour!"

It's not enough in aerobics that you just *do* these hateful exercises. No, you have to act like you're having a really great time while you're doing them. They have this little "Yip" you're supposed to do to show what a gol-darn good time you're having. Every fifteen or twenty seconds someone whose makeup doesn't even run while she's hopping and flopping around will yell, "Yiiiip!" So, I learned the "Yip." Now I just stand in the back and "Yip," and they don't even notice that I'm not doing the routine.

Now, I don't want to cast any aspersions here (my arms are too tired after aerobics to "cast" anything—I couldn't even *roll* an aspersion). I'm definitely not saying all aerobic instructors are not bright. I'm simply saying that I have my doubts about my aerobics instructor due to the fact that she is constantly warning us,"Don't forget to breathe." Like I'm not going to notice after 10 or 15 minutes. (How many funerals have you been to where the deceased had "forgotten" to breathe?)

(Sob) "Oh, if only we'd reminded her to breathe."

"Yes, but she really looks fit, doesn't she?"

Besides, I have a theory that too much exercise actually robs your brain of valuable oxygen. What with all that moving, hopping, and shaking of your extremities, what could be left for your brain? Or, maybe it's those little headbands, choking off the blood supply.

What else besides the premature death of many brain cells, could explain the concept of a triathalon? That's the race in which the addled participants swim two miles, ride a bike for 100 miles, and then run a marathon. It's sometimes called an "Iron Man" contest—no doubt named after the steel plates in the heads of the participants. Even the rigorous, years-long training of a gymnast like Mary Lou Retton took such an obvious toll that she can no longer eat Wheaties without spilling milk all over herself.

Of course, Mary Lou is rich now, what with all those commercials. She even sold her name to Sears for a line of little girls' exercise wear—"Mary Lou Retton Exercise Wear." I have a feeling that even if I get really famous, Sears is not going to buy my name for clothes. For one thing, you need a glamorous image. It's hard to be glamorous when you're so darn short. I'm barely 5'1". You know how they always say those tall "leggy" beauties like Darryl Hannah or Brooke Shields have "legs that just won't quit?" Well, I have legs that won't *start.*

If I were a *Playboy* centerfold (in a "theme" issue of "The Ladies of Comedy" with, for instance, Erma Bombeck, Roseanne Barr, and me), the staple would be in my *ankles.*

I try to keep up with fashion trends despite my size. Like most women in America, I had my "colors" done. You know where they try to determine what "season" you are? I'm a "Hallowe'en". It's a short season. They recommend wearing "black" and "orange" and favor tall, pointy hats.

We Baby Boomers have been harangued about fitness ever since 1960 when Jack Kennedy beat Richard Nixon and strode youthfully to the highest office in the land. Here was a gigantic family constantly involved in some form of activity from sailing at Hyannisport, to tennis, to a rigorous game of touch football. And they wanted all the rest of us to be just as active as they were. (Sadly, of course, later on we discovered that at least some of the "activity" the Kennedy boys were engaging in was kind of *like* touch football—only without the ball.)

My own family was considerably smaller and more sedentary. We did sometimes play a rousing game of "Hide the Thimble," but only the one hiding it got even a semblance of exercise.

Even though I never played touch football, I came to enjoy watching football on TV in the bosom of my all-male family (which included one husband, one son and one formerly male cat). It is a comfort to me that I almost always weigh less than anyone on the football field, with the possible exception of some of those wimpy soccer-style kickers.

I've noticed that men and women have a different attitude toward the game of football. I like to make it a social event. I like to have a few snacks, a few drinks, and then, maybe a few snacks. And if anything happens—which is very rare in the game of football—I watch it on Instant Replay and snack.

But men want to watch every stinking minute. I've found if you yak continuously at your man during a football game, you can get him to promise you almost *anything* to shut up. If you add vacuuming, you can even get a trip to Hawaii. OK, One-Way, alone, but still . . . I've always found a way to get back.

Well, I sincerely hope you are able to integrate exercise into your life. I am unimpressed with the promise that it will extend your life; I think it only *seems* longer. But when I pass on to my eternal reward, I have instructed my heirs to wait about six months to mark my final resting place with this epitaph:

"Here lies Susan Vass, indistinguishable in permanent

repose from her activity level in life. But she finally weighs her ideal weight."

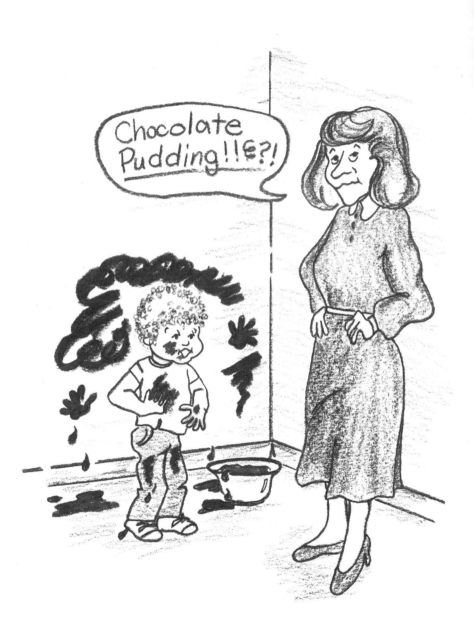

Chapter
3

Laughing Your Way
Through Motherhood

Motherhood is a profound, intense experience. I think your first-born is always the biggest shock to your system—even though you have nine months to prepare for it. I know I spent the whole first week waiting for the parents to come home and pay me!

I wanted to be a mother for as long as I can remember. I got a doll each year for Christmas until I was 14. Still those 14 "children" were mercifully mute at 2:00 a.m. and didn't seem to mind a bit being tossed naked into the toybox until they piqued my interest again.

Real children are a tad more demanding. Not to mention expensive. When my husband and I were newlyweds, we started a "Baby Fund" in an old Marlboro box with a slit cut in the top. Our other little hippie friends would throw spare change in and were quite astonished by our rigorous planning for this as yet unconceived baby. I think at one point we had accumulated upwards of nine dollars before some emergency, like groceries, reared its ugly head and wiped out our fund.

Six years later when we had our baby, it was amazing how expensive miniature t-shirts and pants could be. In fact, there seemed to be an inverse relationship (like, in swim suits) between the amount of cloth and the price. Thank God for baby showers at which we were given so many little "receiving" blankets (a dangerous name, because men sometimes think this means you can "pass" the baby to a wide receiver as long as he is swaddled in a receiving blanket. This is inaccurate.) Also kimonos, and rubber pants and tiny suits that all say "L'il Cowpoke" or "Astronaut" or "Olympian."

I was so fascinated with these tiny garments that I played with them night and day until they got so dingy that I had to wash them. I hung them out on the line to dry and all the neighbors assumed that the baby had been born.

There are many different styles of mothering. My own mother (Saint Dorothy—you may know her) makes Donna Reed look like a slouch. She's right out of a 1950's sitcom complete with housedresses and cobbler aprons, chocolate chip cookies baking and an utterly spotless house. She practices "preventive" cleaning—dusting and vacuuming *before* one dirt or dust molecule can accumulate, washing the dishes *before* we eat—things like that. If you asked her the two greatest contributions to civilization, she wouldn't say "fire" and "the wheel." No, her answer would be "Hi-lex and rubber gloves."

She was my role model and a tough act to follow. She bathed us about eleven times a day. I still blame my dry skin condition on all those early baths.

I saw a slightly different mothering style the other day. A young woman, nine months pregnant on the back of a Harley was wearing a black leather maternity top with BABY spelled out in studs. I don't know for sure, but I *suspect* that her child will not grow up with dry skin.

As little girls growing up, except for our own mommies with all their particular eccentricities, we have very few role models for mothering. The fairy tales have an inexplicable absence of mothers except for "wicked" stepmothers.

Cinderella had no children. Neither did Sleeping Beauty—her name is a dead give-away. And Snow White had no children, although seven short husbands would be a bit of a strain.

Sometimes I feel that I got tricked into becoming a mother by watching *Little House on the Prairie.* Where did they get those kids? Have you ever known any real-life children who were as well-behaved as they were? I can't recall the last time my son called me "Maw" or said "Yes'm" when I asked him to do something. Nor has he tearfully confessed that he sure learned a valuable lesson about doing chores when all the chickens died after not being fed for three days. Of course, we have no chickens, but you get the idea. He has no chores either, even though he is 16. I tried to get him to take out the garbage on Wednesday nights, but he called up the child protection people and asked to be placed in foster home.

It was a big night at the Ingalls' house when Charles Ingalls would take down his fiddle to play for the family. Yes, that would really light up my son's eyes. I can hear his little squeals of delight now:

"I'm sure. Gag me. It's Dad and his totally awesome fiddle again. Get a life!"

It takes a lot more to excite the children of today, doesn't it? Fortunately, nothing that 5 or 10,000 dollars won't buy.

My son wanted to know if Laura and Mary had kerosene video games. All in all, you've got to hand it to the pioneers. It's bad enough to *drive* from St. Joe, Missouri to California. Can you imagine *walking?* Behind an ox? Or, if you were one of the lucky ones to ride in the covered wagon—2,000 miles, no shocks, seven to ten kids, no TV, no Nintendo. Seven to ten kids going, "Moooom, are we West yet?" "How many more miles to the West?"

We drove to Disneyland last year. Four thousand miles in a VW Rabbit with only an AM radio. By the time we got to Anaheim, we didn't have to worry about the much-vaunted freeway shootings so much as about gunfire *within* the car.

But clearly, the whole pioneer family was made of sterner stuff. Caroline Ingalls was no wimp herself. She was always so pathetically excited when Charles would buy her a bolt of cloth for her birthday to make a dress for *herself.*

The only bad apples on The Prairie were Mrs. Olson and her two possessed children, Nellie and Willie Olson. Each week, Nellie or Willie would break something and blame Laura, or cheat in school and blame Laura, or rig the big horse race and blame Laura, or kill the schoolma'rm and blame poor blind Mary. Each week their treachery would be discovered and they would appear to learn a lesson, which would last for precisely six days, until the next episode.

My own son Jacob, while not being overly-ambitious at household chores, is an excellent student. But he's not good in Art. He came home after the last grading period with this green and purple woven basket and he had received a D+ on it. I was pretty peeved, because *I* had done well over half of that thing. I thought it was a darn fine basket. I would like to see the other mothers' baskets.

It took me right back to my own illustrious art career in 7th grade when I received a D+ on a soap carving of a boat, which was actually my third attempt. My art teacher wouldn't accept the first two carvings which were "The Ten Commandments After Moses

Broke Them," and "The Washington Monument," respectively.

Neither could I master "drawing in perspective" nor life-model drawing, although personally I think *my* "Nude Descending a Staircase" was every bit as good as Pablo Picasso's—he just had better P.R.

I wasn't good at Home Economics either—particularly the sewing part. I spent six weeks making a hanky. But I come from a long line of women who couldn't sew. It was tough growing up in the '50's if your mother didn't sew, because there always seemed to be some kind of pageant or recital requiring a costume. How vividly I recall Christmas when I was an angel in the pageant and all the other little girls had the beautiful regulation angel costumes. I had two dish towels stapled together at the shoulders and a wire coat hanger wrapped with tinfoil from the bottom of the oven for a halo. Halloween was kind of a nightmare too. My best friend Kakky had a Tinkerbell outfit, and my friend Mary was a fairy princess. My Mom just handed us all Bibles and sent us out as Jehovah's Witnesses.

In 1969 I attempted to make my husband a Nehru jacket for his birthday. This was an unbelievably ugly green-and-gold paisley garment that enjoyed 20 minutes of popularity when the late Sammy Davis, Jr. wore one on T.V. It took me until 1979 just to do the collar. By the time I finally finished it, even the Goodwill wouldn't take it. They felt that being poor was burden enough on their customers; being poor and looking ridiculous was adding insult to injury.

My son is also a French student. He tells me his French name is "Herve." I remember mine was Michelle. We were assigned these French names and then had to practice saying them for many days. "Bonjour, je m'appelle Michelle." (Hello, my name is Michelle). After about two weeks of this, my friend Bonnie (not the brightest bulb on the Christmas tree), suggested that we were *ready* to go to France. I disagreed. "Bonnie," I said, "I can only say *one thing.* And it's a *lie.*" Then we worked on such valuable phrases as "the pen is on the table." You know, it's remarkable how infrequently that comes up in regular conversation. You have to take the pen to France; you have to put it on the table; then you have to wait for your chance to draw attention to it. Other people are discussing Proust or Descartes, or the value of the franc versus the dollar, and you pipe up, "But, the pen is on the table!" Mighty impressive.

One of the first things that comes up when you have young children is the question of pets. Pets provide excellent training in nurturing, cleaning up after, and feeding them—for the mothers of the children who own them.

So, then the question becomes what kind of pet? Fish are easy to care for, fun to watch, but have notoriously short lifespans. For this reason, I recommend Walleye or Trout. At least they can be eaten if you discover them soon after they croak.

There are numerous fans in the "dog camp" to be sure, but in our series of cramped, cheap, city apartments they were not welcome. When we finally did move to a cramped, cheap house in the suburbs there were all kinds of ordinances governing the ownership of dogs. There is also the matter of paper training, regular outings, walking, etc. And the fact that you can't leave them alone for very long at all. Cats seemed to be a better alternative for our family.

We had a beloved family cat named Tiger. He was an 18-lb. tomcat—kind of a pit cat, really. He was very smart—a sort of feline Einstein. He learned how to jump from the deck, to the lower roof, to the roof of the dormer, and down a narrow stretch of roof to the window of the master bedroom. Then he would knock on the window until it was opened and he would come in, frequently with inert furry friends in his mouth. He would happily roam the house, use his box, and then jump into our bed, playfully, but firmly, swat us in the face and demand to be let out the same window. This he did several times a night and trained us so well that after a few years, we didn't even think it strange. Our own infant son slept through the night at two weeks, so why we put up with letting a large, orange cat in and out seven or eight times a night is still a mystery to us. I guess because we really loved him.

Anyway, as all cats do, he used up his nine lives at the rate of better than one a year, and eventually one very sad July day he went to the great litter box in the sky.

With our minds still numbed with grief, we went down to the Ramsey County Humane Society intending to get another cat. But unfortunately, every one of us picked up a cat and no one would put theirs back. They have a big sign on the wall saying, "We will kill the animals in 24 hours," so you have a huge feeling of responsibility to salvage as many as you possibly can. Later we found out that our teenage son is allergic to cat hair in large quantities. But he's doing great in that foster home now.

So, now we have three cats, which turns out to be against some Cat Quantity Ordinance in our suburb of Maplewood. Cats are also supposed to be "leashed," despite the fact that any leash which is small and tight enough to prevent them from escaping is also, coincidentally, exactly the smallness and tightness necessary to kill them. So, in flagrant violation of our ordinance, we let our cats run free and every few weeks the anal-retentive lawn fetishes in our neighborhood leave anonymous brochures in our mailbox with the leash ordinance highlighted in angry yellow marker. Not for nothing are these types inordinately concerned about "Crab" grass, if you get my drift...

So, anyway, we had these three kittens and I learned a profound truth about them. They are basically babies without diapers. And the carpet in our family room is now a color Sears calls "Desert Sand." You've heard of "Life in the Fast Lane." This is "Life in a Litter Box." One of the three kittens, an exceptionally beautiful tortoise-shell female named Amber, turned out to be a real bimbo—a feline Dan Quayle. It took her six months to master the litter box and my mother, an old farm girl who thinks all cats belong in the barn chasing rodents, wanted to make her into a coat collar.

These cats are very fussy eaters. They will only eat one kind of cat food—Tender Vittles—the expensive kind, of course. And only one flavor of Tender Vittles—Gourmet Dinner. Give me a break. We're talking about an animal that uses its tongue for toilet paper!

That's hardly my idea of a gourmet. And yet that same cat can finish his or her personal hygiene, and turn up its little whisker-laden nose at things named "Savory Supper", "Country Buffet", even "Seafood Delight" because it isn't *good* enough. Heck, some of those things sound so good, I have been tempted to try them.

Last summer the cats brought a huge epidemic of fleas into the house. We had to get the Pest People to come and spray the whole house with gallons of expensive, undoubtedly-carcinogenic liquid. Then we had to bathe the cats in special flea shampoo, cleverly named Scratch-Ex. Take a wild guess who this job fell to? That's right—Mom. Luckily, they had directions on how to do it on the bottle. It started out, "wet cat's hair." Which is a good thing, because I would have forgotten that for sure. Then, "work up a good lather, starting with the head and moving back toward the tail." Now, the next instruction was obviously written by someone who has never known a cat personally: "Allow lather to remain for five minutes"! Have you ever tried to confine three lathered-up cats for five minutes? I wouldn't have thought that an animal that small could rip ceramic tile off a wall...

So, in order to punish them for bringing the fleas into the house—we had them all fixed. Oh, lighten up, I'm only kidding. (But, if you are in a supervisory position, this is an excellent disciplinary tool.)

No, really, it *had* to be done. We had two little girl cats and one little boy cat, so we could see big, big trouble down the road. We had tried the kitty condoms. But these are not responsible animals! And they're very nocturnal. They come to you at three o'clock in the morning, begging for help putting them on. Otherwise they would put holes right in 'em.

So, we had to have the cats fixed. The vet always says the same thing: "The little boy cat will be so much *happier* after he's fixed."

I doubt it. I have known a lot of male persons in my life and when you ask them what would make them really, really happy, rarely do they mention neutering.

Now, some of you might be thinking, "Oh, we liked you a lot Susan, but now you've gone and mentioned condoms." It's not a dirty word, my friends. Not in this day and age. In fact, if you search this whole book through you will not find one "dirty" word, unless you have inadvertently dropped the book in the street on the way home. This, my friends, is not just a book you can *give* your mother: it's a book I have *dedicated* to my mother.

You know, even though parenting sometimes seems like a lot of work, there are surely emotional rewards in abundance. Just a few years ago, my son came home from school with a questionnaire from his Family Living Class. The first question was, "What do you *dislike* about your parents?" and he had written, "they yell at me." I said, "WHY THE HECK DID YOU SAY THAT, IT'S EMBARRASSING?!!" The next question was, "What do you *like* best about your parents?" and I was thinking, "kind, considerate, fun to be around." But no, what does *my* son like best about his parents? "They can drive!" It just gives you that warm-all-over feeling. Makes you want to run right out and procreate again.

Not only are the cats fussy eaters, but my son is really fussy. He's at that stage of teenagehood where he thinks the four food groups are salt, sugar, grease, and a beverage. I went on a speaking tour recently and made up numerous meals in advance for the family. Put some in the fridge, some in the freezer, color-coded them and put the color-coded list on the refrigerator door with a Garfield magnet that says, "Are we having fun yet?"

Well, I get back a few days later and find about 50 Burger King bags spread all over the house, including the bathroom. And in the refrigerator—untouched—is the tuna-noodle casserole. The good one, too, with the peas and the potato chips on top—untouched. With "Mr. Yuk" stickers all over it.

It's very hard to cook for someone whose idea of "fruit" is Cherry

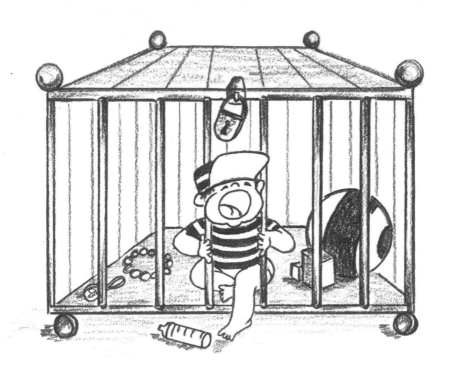

Coke.® Speaking of Coke®, I have fond childhood memories of dividing an 8-oz. bottle (yes, boys and girls, there used to be glass bottles before aluminum cans and plastic bottles which will be with us in toxic waste dumps until roughly 3500 AD.) between my two siblings and me. We would get out these little skinny Tupperware juice glasses and then according to the "Children's Bill of Rights, Third Amendment on Dividing Things Up Among Siblings," one sibling got to do the dividing, and the other got to choose first. Thus great care was taken to get the dividing "even," down to the last Coke® molecule. This process would sometimes take hours. By the time we got it perfectly even, the Coke® was warm and had no fizz, but by God it was fair.

Responsibilities such as Fair Coke® Dividing, Mandatory Younger Sibling Teasing, and Conning Younger Siblings Out of Money (by convincing them that *17* pennies were *way* more money than two lousy *quarters*) weighed heavily on my young life.

People think children have such a soft life, especially babies. But if that's true, why do so many babies deliberately try to kill themselves? Sure they do. If an *adult* put a fork in a light socket, did a half-gainer down the basement stairs and whipped up a nice breakfast of marbles and Chlorox, that person would be taking a mandatory long rest in a state facility for the very, very depressed.

And no wonder babies are depressed. They are in jail most of the day. True, we call it a "crib" or a "playpen," but face it, it's a cage.

Then, look at their boring diet. For breakfast: milk. For lunch: oh lookee, milk again. Dinner? Let's see, how about some NICE MILK! No pizza, no sushi, no Szechuan chicken wings. I'd kill myself too.

Much later, when children can choose their diet, they tend to be drawn to less-than-gourmet items. This accounts for the virus-like proliferation of "family fun" pizza restaurants named after rodents. This is not good training for children's dining out experiences. In 20 years, they will be at a chi-chi restaurant like Sardi's or "21" running between tables wearing funny hats, asking the maitre'd how many tokens you get for pheasant under glass.

The Rodent Namesake Restaurant in my hometown here in Minnesota has a room with a giant 6-foot muppet of Elvis Presley. You put in a quarter and The King sings his big hits. Believe me when I tell you that The King is very ratty-looking. He doesn't look much better than Elvis himself probably looks right now.

Whatever else you say about them, babies are *not* lazy. After several months of being strapped to a board and then a few more months behind bars, they are just bursting with pent-up energy. It's as if they punch a little time clock when they hit the ground running each morning:

> "Okay, gotta take out all these pot lids. There, that's better...Now, let's unroll the toilet paper. Boy, a baby's work is never done...Heck, Mom should buy riper bananas—it's hard work mashing these into the piano keys...uh oh...ten minutes in the penalty box...time to finger-paint on the kitchen wall with chocolate pudding. Hey, who put those pot lids away, now I have to do it all over again! Lunch break!"

Soon enough, children discover board games. The object of any board game is *not* to have fun or while away a few pleasant hours. No, the object of any board game is to win. Children are naturally cut-throat competitors. A seven-year-old boy will play full-contact Chutes and Ladders. But he prefers to play Candyland with the color-blind.

One mistaken notion about board games is that your family will have as much fun playing them as the deranged people in the television ads. I must remind you: these are actors. They are being paid a lot of money to look like they are having a nearly-orgasmic time.

I know this because I have done commercials in which I had to bite a Twinkie and look ecstatic. Ladies and gentlemen, there is, in the elegant world of commercial acting, a thing called a "spit bag" wherein the actor bites the food item, smiles like he or she has just won the Michigan Lottery, and then SPITS THE ITEM OUT in a bag held by an unfortunate called "best boy" or "gaffer" or one of those glamour jobs you always see in the credits of movies.

No one has *ever* had as much fun playing "Spill the Beans," "Uncle Wiggley" or "Careers" as the TV families are having. What will happen when your real family plays "Careers" is one person will be winning and going "hahahahahahahahahaha" to his sibling; one person will be reading a book; and one person will get mad and knock over the Opportunity Cards. Soon after that, a spirited "hands-on" experiment over the ancient philosophical question: "Does physical violence solve anything?" will ensue.

It is also axiomatic that the child who owns the game will win. It's not so noticeable in board games, which are more games of chance, but it's definitely evident in the skill games like ping pong. And forget about video games. No adult on Earth has the hand-eye coordination to take on anyone over the age of four. If Darwin is to be believed, the process of evolution will mandate that the entire next generation of children will be born, not with hands, but with joysticks.

Another thing that always *looks* like more fun than it is, is camping. In Minnesota people are crazy for camping, especially "up North" which is a region near the Canadian border synonymous with Hell, as far as I'm concerned—a place where you cannot find a decent Thai restaurant for hundreds of miles.

I'm not camping until they come up with a Coleman microwave. I'm sorry, but you look up "vacation" in the dictionary, you will not see someone chopping wood to build a fire to boil water to wash the bean juice off tin dishes. No. A "vacation" is lying on a white sand beach while tan, attractive men bring you drinks with umbrellas.

Up North, they do not bring drinks to your campsites; and they don't put umbrellas in beer.

PLUS, the ugliest of God's creatures live in the woods. After the Flood, Noah took all the cute animals like dogs and cats and gerbils and said, "You'll live in houses and eat out of dishes." The *next* cutest—cows, pigs, ducks and such—He said: "You'll live on farms. We'll take turns; first, we'll feed you…and then you'll feed us."

But the truly ugly things like snakes, bears, and mosquitos, mice, bats, and horned owls, He said:

"You go live in the woods and eat each other. If you're real good, and don't go near houses or farms, every once in a while I'll send you some campers."

I have tried to be a sport. I have slept in a moist pup tent that smelled like the inside of a never-laundered gym shoe. Do you know what you always hear in the tent, right before drifting off to an uneasy sleep? *One* mosquito—which sounds like the 101st Airborne.

There is only one thing worse than that sound, and that is when it *stops*. And you know it's somewhere on your body. It feels like a million, trillion mosquitos are everywhere on your body. Finally, you feel the bite and WHACK! You GOT IT! Blessed relief.

Just before your weary eyelids crash, your hear:

"*zzzzzzzzzzzzzzzzzzzzzzzz*. Let's go, Joan, they got Martha."

But at least mosquitos are an insect I understand. They drink your blood to live. It's not their fault, they are just trying to survive. An insect I do not understand is the gnat. You are out for a walk on one of Minnesota's two beautiful summer weekends, and suddenly this cloud of gnats is buzzing all around your head. They don't light; they don't bite. What the heck do they want from me?

Cooking in the Great Outdoors is a separate skill. Hint: Sauerbraten is a bad choice. It has to marinate for three days, during which it will attract the attention of your friendly outdoor animals. Then it has to cook for three hours on your stove at home, or roughly 36 hours over a campfire. Also, the cast-iron, three-quart pot necessary to make the dish will be an unwelcome addition to your husband's backpack.

Going to the bathroom outdoors need not even be discussed here, except to observe that when Freud thought he had detected female "envy" of a celebrated male part, he had probably been talking to Viennese women who had recently been camping.

Just for the record, you should also know that Haagen Dazs keeps very poorly in your standard camping cooler. It all has to be eaten up on the first day of the trip—preferably in the car on the way to the campsite.

If you think summer camping in Minnesota is about as much fun as a date with Morton Downey, you should also know that there is a sport here called "Winter Camping." No, I am not making this up. A demented guy I know named Jack went camping one Christmas Eve, all by himself, up North where he burrowed into a snowbank in his extra-thick winter sleeping bag and listened to the wolves howling all night long. He said it was his most peaceful Christmas ever, a statement he made when we were spending Christmas in *Maui* together, so you figure it out. He is now under serious psychiatric care.

It gives one pause to realize that a baby born today will graduate in the Class of 2007. Just four years after that, my mortgage will be paid off, but that is another story.

It won't be easy to be a kid in 2007. It wasn't really *that* easy to be a kid in 1957, although we tend to remember those days as "Good Olde." Today's children's lives are quite different from what they used to be, a fact which can be demonstrated by examining the four most common excuses for not having your homework done—then and now.

Top Homework Excuses in 1959

1. I left it on the piano.
2. The dog ate it.
3. I was sick.
4. Somebody "died." In college, many of us killed off our entire families numerous times over. The trick was remembering which professor we tearfully told about "Grammy's" demise, and which one we informed about the passing of beloved Uncle George.

Top Homework Excuses Today

1. The computer was down.
2. Aliens took it.
3. I left it at my non-custodial parent's house.
4. I sold it to buy crack cocaine.

Competition for grades has become very keen from the time the "Yuppie Only Children" try to get into the best pre-schools, to the day they are accepted into the college of their choice. It is difficult to avoid being sucked into this grade rat race and you will be sorely tempted to "help" your child with his or her homework.

I know reputable child guidance counselors say it is important to make the child responsible for consequences of behavior such as procrastination.

"You must teach them 'ownership' of their grades," they advise sternly.

I don't *want* him to own a "D" in English. What if he can't get into *any* college—even a community college—and he has to live with us forever and ever?

Thus, when your son informs you at 7:00 p.m. that he has a term paper on "whales" due the *next day*, you can't calmly say "Isn't *that* special?" or words to that effect. No, you hustle him frantically into the car and haul him off to the library where you quickly discover that the whole class has the same assignment. The parking lot is chock-full of Suburban wagons with tight-lipped mothers who are making a beeline for the card catalogue. Any mother who has ever gotten into a physical fight with another mother over the last copy of "Our Friends the Whales," or who has driven 75 miles to a library in a distant suburb knows what I am talking about.

There are, of course, some subjects that you cannot "cram" for. I will never forget the shock I experienced when I realized that in chemistry you cannot read the flyleaf of the chemistry text and give a glib oral report. Do you ever wonder when crossing a bridge whether those engineers "crammed" and have now forgotten as much as you have about Western Civ 101?

In a world where we try to encourage our sons to be "kinder, gentler" males, many of us forward-thinking mothers tried to get our boy babies to like dolls. I bought my son a sweet, soft-bodied baby doll for his second Christmas. He played with her for about 16 seconds, including getting her out of the box. After that, he enjoyed her mainly as a sponge to mop up spilled juice, or as a brief experiment in hairdressing, a profession for which he apparently has scant aptitude. Using only plastic "safety" scissors and a Fisher-Price tool kit, he created the first "punk" haircut in 1974.

Still, things have loosened up a little regarding gender-appropriate toys. When my brother was little, he wanted an Easy Bake Oven in the worst way. My father insisted that it was a "girl" toy. Finally, they got a long extension cord and put it in the backyard and called it an "Easy Grill." He spent many happy hours outside with a chef's hat and a spatula. Because, you see, it's "manly" to do anything as long as it's *outside.*

"Say, isn't that Harold doing needlepoint?"

"Yes, but he's out on the deck, so it's okay."

You can only do needlepoint *indoors* if you're Rosie Greer. If you're a 300-pound man, you can crochet doilies or make pot holders on a loom, and nobody's going to say a word except "Nice doily."

I am probably inching myself out on a stereotypical limb here, but I believe that there is something almost genetic about a little boy's fascination with creepy, crawly, slimy things like spiders, salamanders and toads. I was quite a tomboy myself and loved tree-climbing, sports, and a modest level of good-natured violence, but I never took to snakes or frogs. When my baby brother was barely three years old, he hid a salamander in a magazine, climbed up on my lap with the magazine, and sweetly asked me to read him a story. The magazine fell open to the place where the living bookmark was stuck to the page, and my screams could be heard in the next county.

I think I always felt sorry for the animals when little boys got hold of them, even when they meant them no deliberate harm. Imagine it from the frog's point of view. A particular frog is having a

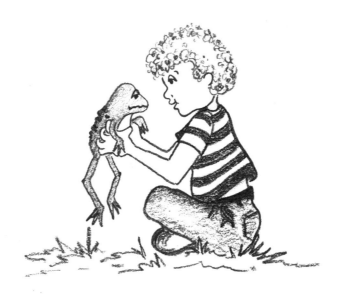

perfectly nice life in a shallow stream, when suddenly a giant, sticky, shrieking lunatic grabs him and thrusts him into a Tupperware bowl with nailholes punched randomly in the lid so that it will *never* "burp" again.

This frog must think it has landed in the Ninth Ring of Hell. And just when he thought life could get no worse, an even *larger* shrieking lunatic—the owner of the former Tupperware—discovers him and blames *him* for his miserable existence in her favorite bowl.

Needless to say, little girls were surely affected by sexist toys. As I have already admitted, I loved dolls. Dishes were okay, too, because you got to slop around in water which all kids love and, as a little girl, you had no idea of the long trail awinding on *that* score. If you *had* known for a minute just how many dishes you would wash in one lifetime, you probably would have done a swan dive right out of your crib.

But, when you got that toy *iron*, you definitely began to suspect that your future wasn't going to be a day at the beach.

The only dolls I did not like were "bride" dolls and Barbie. With a "bride" doll, you had the wedding and that was pretty much the end of it. We weren't nearly as knowledgeable or sophisticated as young girls today, so we didn't know how to play "honeymoon."

Barbie was another kettle of fish. You couldn't very well "mother" a doll whose breasts—even actual size—were larger than your own.

Clearly, then, the sole purpose of Barbie is to dress her. I think Barbie has a pernicious influence on future women. Oh, I'm not talking about the accurate criticism by some feminists that Barbie is anatomically incorrect, that she encourages little girls to become mindless adult consumers, endlessly concerned with surface appearance, or that she requires a wardrobe that rivals the costume department at Warner Brothers. These are minor criticisms.

No, I'm talking about something much more basic here, and that is the notion that here is a woman who stays the same weight her entire life! Putting aside the fact that if Barbie were constructed to scale, the lifesize version would measure 58-22-34, her main crime is that she never gains an ounce. This raises entirely unrealistic expectations in female persons.

Where is the Preggers Barbie who swells up like a balloon and has chunky, edemic ankles? Where is the Dieting Barbie who has three complete wardrobes: size 10 Calvins, roomy shifts, and small pup tents? Where is Barbie's exercycle to sit and gather dust in the basement of her dream house? Where are the latex stretch marks on her little rubber thighs from 23 diets in the last seven years?

More than enough said.

One thing is certain—a baby of either sex loves blankets. The kind with satin binding you can feel while you suck your thumb or twist your hair. Blankies provide such warmth and security, I wonder why we ever give them up. I wish I had mine right now.

My son's blanket was called, for reasons we never determined, Waddie. *Everyone* called it his "Waddie"—babysitters, grandpar-

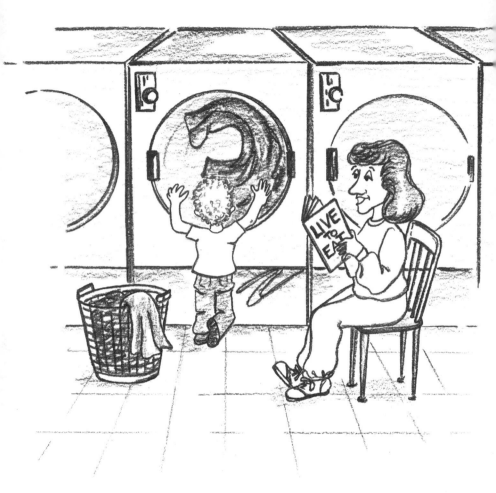

"Waddie" is not dead.

ents, and of course, we, his parents. He also called bread "ba," so that two otherwise quite intelligent grownups would have conversations like this:

"Have you seen Jacob's Waddie? It's almost nap time."

"I last saw it under his highchair. Please pass the ba."

Waddie was a soft, light, loose-woven thermal blanket with the obligatory satin binding. Waddie was mint green. One day Waddie disappeared, an event roughly on a par with the sun not rising. I raced to the little "dime" store (apparently named when you could still buy something for a dime) from whence Waddie had originally come. Alas, there was a Waddie-like sibling, identical in every respect except for its color, which was PINK. In desperation, I bought it and it became New Waddie. New Waddie was decidedly different, but Jacob took it pretty well. Then, miraculously, Old Waddie showed up (proving once again, that you *should* clean behind the stove), so we thought we had a back-up.

Except, of course, now he had to have *both* Old and New Waddies at nap time, bed time, or travel time.

Waddie could not be laundered with any regularity, for it altered the item in some way known only to a two-year-old—probably smell. After a decent interval of being wet upon, spilled upon, and dragged across floors that, charitably, did not resemble the pristine Congoleum in *House Beautiful,* I would wrestle Waddie from Jacob's trembling fingers and spirit it off to the laundromat where he would carefully monitor each spin of the dryer until it emerged a cleaner, brighter, if slightly-defective, Waddie.

And then he would commence to restoring it to its familiar condition.

He finally and definitively parted with Waddie in second grade, an act I found both sad and brave. I think the world would be a much safer place if we all still had Waddies. Air traffic controllers should have their screens, headsets, and little blankies with wings embroidered on them.

Summit conferences could have the round table, glasses of water, translators and headsets, and President Bush with his red, white, and blue blankie with an eagle on it, and Mr. Gorbachev with a red blankie with a hammer and sickle on it.

Because New and Old Waddies had to travel everywhere, we needed an even larger diaper bag than the one we had received at the baby shower, even though it was larger than some of our early apartments. A diaper bag is designed to cover every possible contingency, a veritable "home away from home" for mother and baby.

For a one-hour outing to a Minnesota park in July, our diaper bag routinely contained:

> 47 Pampers (Regular and Toddler size in case he grew during the outing).
> Gerber Baby Cookies
> Apple Juice
> Orange Juice
> 3 complete changes of outfit
> A $46 pair of useless little Nikes bought because they were "so cute."
> Old and New Waddies
> 11 stuffed toys
> A selection of books, possibly, *The Fuzzy Duckling*, *The Shy Kitten*, and *Green Eggs and Ham*
> A snowsuit and mittens (always a good precaution in Minnesota in July)
> A plastic "changing pad"
> Extra safety pins with plastic duckie heads on them in case the Pamper tabs break
> Baby Powder
> Baby Cream
> Baby Oil
> #30 Sunscreen
> Desitin
> A blanket to sit on
> A pail and shovel
> A couple of playmates

Finally, it is important to pack a couple of "Romance" novels for Mom, books with titles like "Wind-Swept Desires" or "Desirable Sweeping Winds" in which the scantily-clad woman on the cover has a name like Esmeralda or Danielle. If you find a Bertha, a Gladys, or even a Susan in a romance novel, I'll buy you lunch.

Mom needs these romance novels badly, because once a baby arrives on the scene, romance is pretty much shot. Oh, you pretend it isn't, but you're deluding yourself. There isn't even a remote chance that some enchanted evening you may find a sitter. How much romance can you pack in from 8-9:00 p.m. when the only sitter you could find on a school night was an 11-year-old boy with an earring?

Upbeat parenting magazines contain hilarious articles about "Romance After Children." They sternly advise: "Put a lock on your bedroom door!" Like this is going to do it. Any reasonably intelligent 3-year-old has that Fisher-Price hacksaw in the tool kit. And, even if you are blessed with a slow one, there's nothing quite like the piteous bleating of "Mooooom, Mooooom" accompanied by loud door-banging to really get you in a romantic mood.

Once your child enters school, from Kindergarten until senior class pictures, he or she will come home with the same order form for school photos. These photos are traditionally taken in the first week of October, approximately three or four weeks after the start of the school year and offer three "packages" to choose from:

A. **EMBARRASSING:** Which contains four postage-stamp size photos and tells the whole world that you think "upwardly mobile" is something you hang over a baby's crib.

B. **THE TROUBLEMAKER:** This package has 10 wallet photos, 2 5x7's and only *one* 8x10 so the Grandmas will fight over it.

C. **EXTRAVAGANZA:** This package costs enough to feed a family of 4 in Guatemala for a week. It has more "exchange" photos than the number of friends your child will have in his or her whole life.

By the time these pictures are delivered in May, they will not resemble your child in the least.

Boys over the age of eight do not smile for these photos. Usually they will affect the expression of a midget mass murderer. In my son's first-grade picture, his naturally curly hair is wildly askew (á la early pictures of Jerry Rubin or Art Garfunkel). His hair was combed before he left the house, but the hood on his parka messed it all up. He had to wear his parka because it was "the cold season" in Minnesota (October-July). And because he had been up watching his favorite show—*David Letterman*—and had retired at an hour some would find extreme for a six-year-old, he also had dark circles under his eyes. The total effect is rather like an understudy for Linda Blair in *The Exorcist.*

My child happens to be an only child. I did not plan it that way, but that is the way it worked out. Like so many things, there are advantages and disadvantages to this status. I was fortunate to have one sibling of each sex, a sister and a brother. In the Sixties, it was fashionable to issue political statements exhorting the nations of the world to treat each other "like sisters and brothers."

Who are they kidding? Clearly, the proponents of such a plan never *had* sisters and brothers. My sister used to rip the heads off my favorite paper dolls, and once his testerone kicked in, my younger brother used to grab me and practice his wrestling holds. I do not want these examples held up to other nations like China or Iran.

Besides, there are too many nations for each to have a "window seat" on long car trips, and this always leads to trouble.

As a parent, I am admittedly, the world's worst disciplinarian. I consider "I didn't feel like it," to be a fine excuse for why my son didn't do something he was told to do. Perhaps this is because I remember all too keenly the many times when *I* "didn't feel like it," and still don't.

Given this lax attitude, I am very fortunate to have had a child who required very little disciplining. We would "reason" with him until he convinced us of the error of our ways and we gave up. From this "discipline," he has learned persistence and patience with his mental inferiors.

In essence, my parenting approach has been a whole lot of love combined with a careful balance of threats and bribes.

I have read many fine "how-to" guides to communicating with your children. The problem here is that the *child* does not read these books, and consequently does not know the pat little "script" that the author uses as an example.

Sample Dialogue

Mother: "Your cousin Gwendolyn will be coming by for a few hours after school tomorrow. I know you're not too fond of Gwen, but I would really appreciate it if you would try to play with her while your Uncle Charlie runs some errands."

Child: "It's true that I don't like Gwen much because she dropped my cat from the attic window to see if he would land on his feet. But, I will play with her and be especially kind because I think she has low self-esteem."

Real Conversation with Child

Mother: "Your cousin Gwendolyn will be coming by for a few hours after school tomorrow. I know you're not too fond of Gwen, but I would really appreciate it if you would try to play with her while your Uncle Charlie runs some errands."

Child: "Gwen sucks. I'm going to drop *her* from the attic window and see if she lands on her feet."

The teenage years are a great challenge. About the best thing that can be said for them is that your male child will have a renewed interest in intense personal hygiene after a period (ages 8-12) when the only way you could get him to shower was to strap him to the hood of the car and run him through the car wash.

At about 13 my son decided that the entire world was a bleak and terrible place. Also boring. He felt compelled to share these views—via body language, facial expressions, and other nonverbal communication—with everyone who crossed his path, a kind of Johnny Appleseed of Despair.

He is 16 now and is decidedly more optimistic, due in large part to the possession of a driver's license from the naive and trusting State of Minnesota.

Teaching your child to drive is a leap of faith tantamount to that leap of faith required to take off the last industrial-strength Huggie and put on training pants. At some point, it just has to be done. Similarly, you have a $16,000 vehicle, your only child at the helm, and you realize you cannot stay in the church parking lot indefinitely. Sooner or later you must allow him to take the car out onto the street, and months later, the freeway.

Try to be both calm and specific. Say, for example, "Veer to the right to avoid that oncoming truck," rather than "Eeeeeeek, we're all gonna die!"

When your child takes Driver's Ed, he or she will suddenly become a real expert on some of the "basics" you may have forgotten in your everyday driving, like the concept of "signaling your turn." Any experienced driver knows that "signaling" will only inflame the drivers behind you and encourage them to speed up so that you cannot make your lane change.

When my son was a little boy, he always preferred riding with me rather than his father. His father, a very nice man, is also an attorney, and consequently, somewhat of a drag. He doesn't think it's amusing to enter a freeway down an exit ramp in reverse. Children will get a big kick out of this.

Well, this is about all I have to say on Motherhood for the moment. There are numerous areas—from the breast-vs.-bottle controversy to potty-training; from sex education to college entrance exams—that I realize I did not cover. But, I have to save *some*thing for a second book should there be a groundswell movement to that effect.

Just remember to love your children with all your heart, for they are ours for but a little while: 6 years of pre-school, 12 years of school, 4 years of college, 5-10 years of post-graduate work, and 2-5 years of finding themselves before entering the hurly-burly, dog-eat-dog, world of work. Not to mention returning with their children between marriages. So, enjoy.

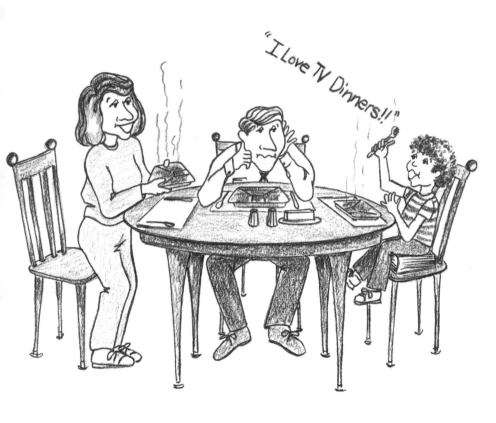

Chapter
4

Laughing Your Way Through Housework & Domesticity

First of all, let me tell you about our house. We bought our first and only house 10 years ago. The realtor, a perky, prevaricating blonde, called it, optimistically, our "starter house." In truth, it almost finished us.

Some jobs are useful to society because they provide employment for sectors that would otherwise be dependent on the dole. For instance, the job of writing copy for real estate ads provides useful work for pathological liars. This has been true probably since the beginning of time when a caveperson ad writer described a 3'x5' cave as "cozy." Crystal Cave—with long pointy stalagmites every two feet—was undoubtedly originally sold as a "handyman's special."

Real estate agents are in a class by themselves, mostly because nobody will sit with them. "Agent" is really a code word for "Great Big Jerk." Witness all the unseemly occupations that have the word Agent attached to them: ad agent, insurance agent, talent agent, FBI agent, and, of course, Agent Orange.

Our dream house was built in 1946 by the architectural firm of Amityville and Usher. We should have been suspicious when the model home was The House That Dripped Blood.

The mortgage has been sold five times in the last ten years. I think now we make our checks out to Guido's Mortgage and Jukeboxes.

What a joy it is to own a home! We keep the heat at 68° as the energy-savers recommend. Actually, that's more of an average. It's 88° upstairs and 48° downstairs. It is very comfortable on the landing. We have our TV there now and we've made it into a tiny family room.

We didn't realize it would be so cold. The FHA certified that the house had an "R38" insulation rating which was at least a strong B+ grade-wise. Little did we know they counted the bat-poop in the attic as insulation. We didn't even know about the bats.

My father, quite the home handyman, has informed us that our house is "settling." Apparently, this is not as good in houses as it is in people. For example, "We are so happy that Joe Bob is finally 'settling' down." With our house, however, it means that the foundation is sinking lower and lower into the ground, until in a few years our only hope will be to sell it as an "earth-sheltered" dwelling.

My sister, Vicki, has the knack of taking an ordinary living space, and even many a dreadful inner-city apartment, and creating a lovely environment with green plants, breezy curtains, a tasteful vase ("voz," not a "vace" which is all I own), an antique photograph, and voilá! A terrific home! She clearly inherited ALL of the cooking and decorating genes, leaving me with the ordering take-out and hiring someone else genes.

The over-all decorating theme of our house and all our previous apartments could best be described as early grad student. During Pre-Lims. We are three Oscars in search of a Felix.

I'm not a very good cook either. I went to *Kramer vs. Kramer* four times just to learn how to make French toast. My favorite ways of consuming food are, in descending order: dining out, take-out, having something delivered, boiling in a bag, and, if desperate, opening a can. This last choice is worst since it involves doing dishes later in the month.

We eat a LOT of frozen dinners. I will pass along this tip to you: never think you can save money by purchasing a "bargain brand" frozen fried chicken. You can't even tell what the pieces *are*. They all look alike, and there's no recognizable shapes like "drumstick" or "wing." You can't even tell if it's light or dark meat. It's all beige.

Not that I am a gourmet. I don't know whether red or white wine should be served with peanut butter and jelly sandwiches. I think it depends on the color of the jelly.

Holidays are a particular strain on bad cooks. Rather than desiccate another turkey, I now make meat loaf in the *shape* of a turkey. If you start when the kids are young enough, they don't know the difference. Much like starting baby puppies out on the 100-lb.

bags of cheap, dry dog food before they learn to like the 89¢ tins of Gourmet Ground Prime.

We don't eat many vegetables in our family. My son has the kind of body that won't tolerate nutrients. But, I do wonder what ad agency really believed that BIRD's EYE was an attractive name for frozen vegetables?

One of the great joys of suburban homeownership is being Up Close and Personal with the wretched refuse of the animal kingdom, like bats, carpenter ants, termites, racoons, and wasps which build their nests in the foundation of your home. One summer and fall we were overrun by these wasps.

We were perfectly happy to *share* our home with them, spending as we did, very little time inside our basement foundation. But they weren't satisfied with sharing. They wanted to come upstairs and watch TV. I can tell you first-hand that wasps are really stupid insects. Hundreds of them fried to death in our dining room light fixture. They would be attracted to the blazing wattage, come too close, and like airheads who fall asleep in tanning booths, would find themselves cooking, and unable to pull away.

This is where the really appallingly low level of intelligence comes in: wouldn't you think, if you were buzzing around a hot light fixture and saw a veritable Wasp Jonestown—that you'd say to yourself, "Ooops, big trouble here, I think I'll go elsewhere."

But no, they'd fly right in there and jockey for space at Armagedden. Wasps are also utterly devoid of social conscience. Sometimes one wasp would be mid-roast and another one would fly in and not once did a roastee try to warn the newcomer:

"Turn back! You're gonna die!"

The wasps stayed in the light fixture for several months because I couldn't bring myself to look at the carnage. They formed kind of a natural dimmer switch which was quite romantic if you didn't look up. Eventually, we had to pay the pest control people (Their motto is: of course it's perfectly safe, just cover all your foodstuffs and leave the house for two days...) to come out and make a surgical strike into the nest itself which turned out to be more efficient than barbecuing them one at a time.

You may be gathering that I am not a good housekeeper, and you would be right on the money. During the last movie I went to, a message came on the screen that said "We have tried to assure our patrons the same comfort and cleanliness of their own home," and I thought "Can't they do any better than *that?*"

I am a person who has moved dirty dishes to a new apartment. I usually decide what I'm going to wear in the morning by what I step on first. My mother, bless her heart, says I find housework be*neath* me, which is not true... I find it be*yond* me.

I don't know how I got to be such a slob, really, because my sainted mother is an incredible housekeeper, as I have mentioned in an earlier chapter.

When company was coming, Mom would clean behind the water heater in the basement. She used to wash all the little Monopoly houses and hotels. She can't stand messes. She cleaned out the attic and threw out all this dusty, fuzzy pink paper, which, sadly, turned out to be the insulation.

So spotless is her house that there is an expression, alas not an *original* one, that people use about her: "Dorothy's so clean," they say, "you could eat off her floors." I'd love to have all the neighbors over, and just have five little piles of spaghetti right there on the floor.

"Come on in, ladies, we're eating off Dorothy's floors. Kick that

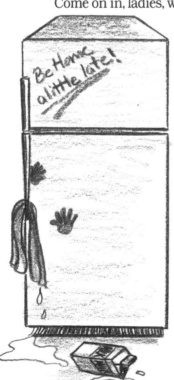

garlic bread over to Dolores, will you please, Bernice?"

Speaking of expressions, here is one Mother herself uses. I was visiting her home in Alexandria, Minnesota, and she had made a big turkey dinner at noon. Along about 7 p.m. we still hadn't had any supper yet and I asked, "Mom, can I give you a hand? What's for supper?"

And she said (here comes the expression): "Oh, honey, we have to eat up this beef. IT'S GOING TO GO BAD."

Yummy! Give me a big slab of that "beef going bad." How do we know we got it in time?

You do learn a lot when you're a lousy housekeeper. I know for certain that none of us is allergic to house-dust, or he or she would be quite dead.

I'm just glad they don't put expiration dates on cleaning products. I don't want Mom coming to visit, picking up my Comet and seeing: AUGUST 1962.

"Oooh, honey, you don't use a lot of *this*, do you?"

Like a lot of families, we leave notes for each other on the refrigerator. Unlike a lot of families, we don't have any magnets. We just write in the dirt and grease on the refrigerator.

Moreover, when you don't do dishes for a week, it can help settle arguments:

"What do you *mean* 'meatloaf again'? Look at these dishes—yesterday we had chicken, the day before that macaroni and cheese, and sometime in the recent period, we must have had either chili or spaghetti, I can't tell which from this plate..."

One housekeeping task that seems particularly pointless is making the beds. My mother says, "Honey (have you noticed she *always* calls me honey?), an unmade bed looks so untidy. What if people see this?"

The way I feel is that if gobs of people are traipsing through your *bedroom*, maybe poor housekeeping is not the most pressing problem in your marriage.

Some things about housekeeping I simply don't understand. Why, for example, do vacuum cleaners have lights? The saleslady says, "It's to see the dirt."

I don't want to see dirt, that's why I'm vacuuming. Besides, anything you can see, it won't pick up anyway. Like the turkey carcass the dog dragged into the bathroom—will it get that? I think not. There's got to be a reason for this light. I think it's this: you're home alone; you hear an intruder; you don't have a flashlight. You whip out the vacuum cleaner, all three of its watts blazing, and shout, "WHO'S THERE?"

Or maybe it's for reading in bed. A way to go blind *and* deaf at the same time.

When you are a really dreadful housekeeper, after awhile you don't notice things. They just become part of the landscape. Like the toenail clipper on the toaster—you pick it up every month, dust it, and put it back.

My mother thinks that because I am such a determined non-cook that I should get a microwave.

"Honey," she says, "not only are they good for 'instant' foods, but microwaves are great when you have forgotten to thaw the meat."

Hey, I own a dryer.

I wish I had the same affinity for green plants as my sister. Her house is so full of greenery, you half expect her husband to come swinging downstairs on a vine. I have slowly killed every single plant

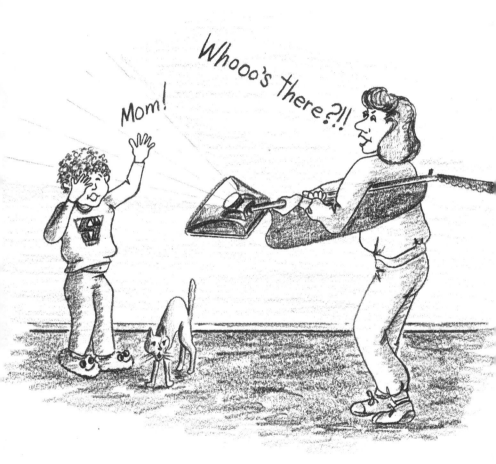

I have ever owned. Silk flowers wilt in my presence. I once spent $300 on a fake tree from a pricey major department store. Two weeks later, all the leaves were on the floor.

Neither do I have an affinity for crafts. I take quite seriously the Biblical admonition: "Consider the lilies of the field. Neither do they toil nor do they spin; yet Solomon in all his glory is not arrayed as one of these."

And so, I neither toil or spin, nor fashion things out of pipe cleaners; nor doth I save old bleach bottles or 5-quart ice cream pails to make clever or decorative household items.

Once I attempted to make Mom a basket out of Popsicle sticks for Mother's Day. I got as far as eating the 173 Popsicles in order to accumulate the sticks. (You know, Popsicles just don't taste as good when you're 38 as when you're 6.)

Each family has someone who's just great at gift-wrapping. In our family, that's Aunt Jessie. Whenever people get a gift from her, they say, "Oh, that's just *too* pretty to unwrap."

When people get a gift from *me* they say, "I think it's so nice when families let the children help."

I want to know if this happens to you, or is only my house possessed? Why didn't they tell us in Science class that the combination of wrapping paper, carpeting, and Scotch Brand Magic Mending Tape creates a force field that attracts half the hair on the planet? Weird hair, too. Hair you've never seen before. Hair in colors nobody in your house has. Hair that gets all *over* the Scotch-Brand Magic Mending Tape and gets permanently imbedded in the package, looking really gross.

Christmas is a time when the clever Craft Queens really shine and klutzes such as myself are embarrassed. My friend Sandy has every square inch of her house decorated—even (I am not making this up) Christmas toilet paper! She has four trees. I always buy a tree that looks like the homely cousin of that motley tree Charlie Brown buys in the 12,345th rerun of "Charlie Brown's Christmas." Then, because I am seriously stature-deficient, I pile all the decorations and lights around the bottom six branches, making the tree look like a festive topless dancer.

This year, we decided to have more of a traditional old-fashioned Christmas. We went out and cut down our *own* tree. It kind of ticked off the neighbors...

One of the worst tasks in the world is taking down the tree. It's not difficult to understand why they call them pine NEEDLES. You could drain spaghetti in your hands when you're done. Do what I do—throw out the whole thing every year. Lights, balls, tinsels, the star—out the door. It's great for the economy. Either that, or wait until Labor Day to dismantle it. It's a lot easier to get the decorations off when *all* the needles are gone.

Whichever course you elect, you've got to vacuum up all the needles and tinsel afterward. Another little tip: if you empty your vacuum cleaner bag and the tinsel is all mixed up with Easter grass, it's probably been too long since you vacuumed.

Housework is a never-ending road to an extremely temporary destination. Imagine driving to California from Miami, staying 15 minutes, and turning around to drive back. Cleaning your house when you have small children is much like shoveling your driveway during a blizzard.

There is a reason we can't keep up. You see, for generations, housework was considered a Woman's full-time job. Our mothers dusted, waxed, polished, swept, mopped, vacuumed, cooked, baked, scrubbed, laundered, ironed, and volunteered, pretty much from sun-up to sun-down. Women worked very hard and were usually supported financially by another person, generally a man, who left the house to go to a paying job.

Nobody asked the Woman, "Do you work?"

If they had, the Woman would have looked very bewildered, not to mention, annoyed.

"Of course I work," she might have said, "How in blazes do you think my family eats?"

This system lasted from c. 11,000 B.C. until the mid-to-late 20th Century when "the people who decide these things" up and reclassified this job and made it part-time.

Now Women "work" all right. And THEN they come home and cook, bake, iron, launder, dust, wax, vacuum, polish and mop.

Some people think the new system is better—some don't. Many have no choice. Some think a new, improved, hybrid system encompassing all of women's reality has to be created.

This New Woman (she even has a magazine named for her) has been called Superwoman, in my opinion, a laughable comparison. What did the *real* Superwoman do, anyway? She flew around rescuing people and beating up bad guys. Do you see her trying to find decent day care for her baby? Do you see her trying to starch her cape and get it pressed for the next day of rescuing? Do you see her putting pork chops in the crockpot before going off to a hard day of beating people up? Do you see her trying to do aerobics on her lunch break so Superman won't run off with Super*girl?* No, she doesn't have to do any of these things. The real Superwoman is a spoiled wimp by comparison.

Part of our problem with housework is trying to match our performances to the pictures in the glossy women's magazines. Ladies, I hate to disillusion you, but these are not *real* people. They do not exist. You can tell by their refrigerators. They always have a whole roasted turkey *and* a ham in there.

When was the last time you had a whole *cooked* turkey in your fridge? What happened? Did she cook the turkey and then nobody showed up for Thanksgiving dinner, not even her husband and children? Did they all disappear into an episode of *The Twilight Zone?* Perhaps her family likes their Thanksgiving turkey cold right from the start, but that seems unlikely.

And ham too? Most people will hardly eat *one* meat any more, let alone two.

Across the page from the standard open-refrigerator ad is a kitchen where *everything*, even the children, look acrylic. There is not one scuff mark or cigarette burn on the floor which is polished more brightly than a boy's first car. There is a table set with unchipped china, crystal water goblets, linen tablecloths, flowers and candles and this is for a simple little supper with the family. There is not *one* jelly glass or plastic Star Wars tumbler from Burger King. And no one with half a brain would put lighted candles on the table for a meal with children, unless they wanted the linen tablecloth set on fire.

Needless to say, my table "settings" are considerably less formal. Often, there are several clean utensils for each person. They may be bunched together on one side of the plate, depending on my energy level and the menu. Who needs utensils for tacos except a big communal spoon to scoop up the meat? The notion of the knife on the right, the spoon next to it, and the fork (or 3 or 4, depending on your income and/or level of pretension) on the left, is pure convention, anyway. Who made these rules and what are the consequences for breaking them? Were people that stupid that, if the fork were on the right and the spoon on the left, they couldn't find them?

I imagine that prehistoric Woman had her hands full with hoping the menfolk would find a nice caribou, skinning the caribou, roasting it over a spit, garnishing it with a little wild parsley, and getting it on what passed for a table to worry too much about whether the gourd went on the right and the arrowhead on the left.

Thankfully, we no longer have to wait for the menfolk to go out and hunt something down for supper, because we now have supermarkets. In some regions of the country, mine being right up there, some men have not assimilated this late-breaking news and persist in dressing in bright orange clothing, grabbing a weapon and heading into the woods to "shop" for meals. Better they should just strap a nice standing rib roast onto the hood of the car and be done with it. But, then they would have to lay off all the nice people who make bright orange clothing, so who am I to complain?

Even grocery shopping can be quite an adventure, although we do not need to wear orange clothing, unless it is "sample day." On this particular day, shoppers roam aimlessly like lethargic herds of cattle from display to display, shoving and pushing and generally making it very difficult to pick up a simple loaf of bread and half-gallon of milk.

Remember: it is up to the supermarket to determine what *is* and what *is not* a sample. Do not think that you can open a package of filet mignon and ask the nice sausage sample lady to throw it on her Hibachi.

Although I consider myself a generally compassionate person, it is my fondest wish that the guy who decided "double bagging" was no longer necessary will someday be buried in a single bag and have the pall bearers try to carry him—and a dozen eggs—to his final resting place. Good luck and godspeed.

I believe that there is a special place in the Not-So-Great Beyond for him and all the people who crash the "10 Items or Less" lane with a cart full of groceries and a sheepish look.

"I know I have six cartons of Coke®, but I thought that should count as *one* thing, you know, cuz like, it's all Coke®. Okay, and the lettuce, cucumber, sprouts, radishes, croutons, French Dressing, avocado, carrots and tomatoes I count as one general thing—SALAD—Okay? And then..."

In addition to the alleged "Express" lane where easily one-third of the customers will have fewer than the maximum number of items allowed, there are usually anywhere from five to 10 other lanes in your regulation supermarket. The law of averages alone would dictate that every fifth to 10th time, *I* would not pick the slowest lane. However, this is not the case. I can pick the lane with only three people in it, while all the others have 22 people, but it turns out, *each* of those 22 people is paying cash or swiftly writing out pre-approved checks, while *my* two people have known the cashier since grade school and have 36 years to catch up on or are trying to cash third-party checks using an outdated library card as an I.D.

The same thing happens at the bank, particularly in the drive-through lines. Things are progressing at a nice clip until the guy ahead of me, in the rusted-out '73 Mercury, attempts to negotiate a three million dollar loan using the car as collateral.

Well, I don't want you to think I am a dead loss at everything domestic. I happen to be very good at laundry. Laundry is a most satisfying chore, with a definite beginning and end. When I was a new bride, I seriously took the advice on the detergent box to "separate things by color." I did all the reds, blues, greens, whites, yellows, etc.—all separately. Sometimes as many as 15 or 20 loads of three items each. Later I realized this was unnecessary; and later still, I washed *every*thing together which created some very nice pink underwear for my husband.

For many years, we lived in apartments which had no laundry facilities, so we had to use laundromats. Leaving home and being forced to guard your laundry lest some unfortunate should steal it from the dryer was, of course, boring and time-consuming. We used to wait until we had a big enough heap that we had to rent a small U-Haul. Often, when we ran out of underwear we would simply buy more. Eventually, however, the trek was unavoidable. Then we would go through all our pockets and seat cushions on a great dime and quarter hunt.

We would descend on the laundromat like terrorists occupying a building, commandeering as many washers at one time as we could without being killed by other patrons. The dryers were massive and signs were posted saying that they could accommodate up to three washer-loads of laundry. However, the temperature of the dryers must have been a balmy 46°, because it took a *roll* of dimes to get the clothes even as far as "damp." One dime lasted about three spins.

When we moved into our house, we had to buy our very own washer and dryer. Imagine my surprise when I went into the basement with a pocketful of change and there was *no place* to put quarters and dimes. It certainly was the dawn of a bright new era for me.

The one irritating part of doing laundry is, no matter how rigorously I check all the pockets of every garment, somehow I *always* wash Kleenex. We all got so used to seeing tiny shreds of Kleenex in all our clothes, that now I just keep a box in the laundry room and throw one in on general principles. Never use white Kleenex after Labor Day.

The universal problem of socks disappearing into the Twilight Zone has been dealt with most thoroughly and humorously by Erma Bombeck and many other comics; nonetheless, it continues to be a great problem at our house. We think it may have something to do with the soaring divorce rate, part of the mad trend of coupled up things in the universe to become single. We do have a reconciliation basket filled with—I am not making this up—over 40 single socks waiting for their mates to turn up again. I think it is hopeless; obviously, they have all run off with younger socks.

Once my laundry is done, I have peaked chore-wise for the week. Ironing follows laundry as dieting follows a binge. In the late 60's and 70's clothes were made primarily of petroleum-based products and did not need ironing. With the trendy return to "natural" fabrics such as rayon and cotton, ironing has made a dramatic comeback as well.

Ironing is a lonely, exacting business. Additionally, it can be a shattering experience emotionally. Here's why: you think of yourself as a clean person. You shower regularly, use deodorant. People don't generally back away when they see you coming. But, every once in a

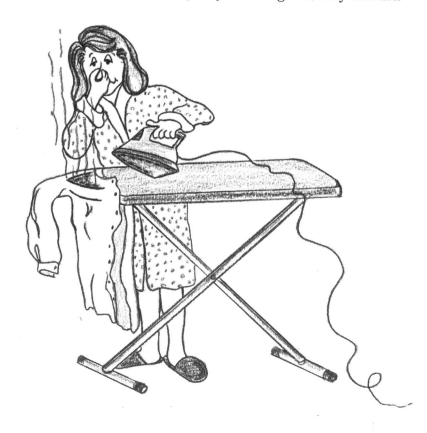

while, when you are ironing, you hit the armpit of a favorite old garment with the tip of that steam iron and a little malodorous cloud wafts up to assault your nostrils.

"Hey," you think, defensively, "who let Hulk Hogan wear this silk shirt?"

When I was a new bride, I used to iron everything—sheets, pillowcases, blue jeans, hankies. My husband stopped asking me to iron his shorts. Right after he explained that he *didn't* mean while he was wearing them.

Now, I iron the absolute minimum. Let's just say that I can't remove my suitjacket without inviting ridicule.

Frequently, I decide that I am going to become a whirling dervish of a housecleaner, that my entire house is going to be organized and spotless. Usually these attacks hit around the first of a new year or on an odd Monday when I find my shoes sticking to the kitchen floor and decide that "THIS IS REALLY IT!"

I start out with a ludicrously grandiose master plan and then stall out when I have accomplished some time-consuming, but ultimately worthless part of the project. Thus, my shoes *still* stick to the kitchen floor but the *spices* are alphabetized.

Because my organizational abilities are much more highly developed than my actual cleaning skills, I do enjoy tasks like rearranging the medicine cabinet, even in a bathroom where, clearly, this is not the highest priority. A bathroom, for instance, in which the shower curtain has become a giant mildew motel. A bathroom in which *the soap* is dirty.

When last I organized the medicine cabinet, I noticed a perplexing caveat on the bottle of my old familiar remedy designed specifically for menstrual cramps.

"Don't take this if you are pregnant," it advised.

Golly, where were *those* people during sex education?

Of course, the tablets were packed in those awful "child-proof" bottles, called this because only a child has hands small enough to align the stupid arrows and pry them open. But "child-proofing" is only the beginning of the frustration.

One nut in Chicago tampers with some Tylenol and suddenly the entire over-the-counter drug industry designs bottles that are virtually impregnable. This particular cramp pill comes in a bottle sealed with cotton, covered with tinfoil, and stuffed into a glued-down box. Then the whole works is shrink-wrapped in plastic. By the time you get it open, your period is over.

Men are at a particular loss with this kind of hysterical

security-conscious packaging because they lack the two things most useful to getting into them—fingernails and patience. There's nothing more pathetic than the sight of a grown man with a bottle of St. Joseph's Aspirin and a chainsaw.

Moving right along in the cabinet, I came to my large celebrity perfume collection. Even though I was valedictorian of my high school class, it still comes as an unpleasant surprise to me when I am wearing Liz Taylor's "Passion" perfume that my eyes do not turn violet. Not once has anyone gotten a whiff of that scent on me and mistaken me for Liz. Cher has a new perfume called "Uninhibited." Shirley MacClaine has one called "Uninhabited."

Then there are the dozens of tubes of lipstick that looked very attractive on my wrist in the store, but looked wretched on my actual face in the cold fluorescent light of day.

Do you know what I think would be a really tedious, stressful job? Naming lipstick colors. Every single year, sometimes more than once, Revlon and L'Oreal and all their cosmetic colleagues reissue the same 67 shades of red, pink, and orange and *some*body has to think up clever new names like "Iced Watermelon" or "Passion Pink."

I bet somewhere in America there is a wild-eyed woman in a rubber room twisting her hair and muttering "Pink Floyd!" "Red Menace!" "Boring Orange!"

A few more random thoughts while puttering in the cabinet:

1. Call it my hang-up if you will, but I believe there is no way to use a rectal thermometer on a child without feeling like a weirdo. Actually, it is not necessary to own any thermometer. Any child who will voluntarily nap *has* a fever.

2. Nair is an unwise alternative to the painstaking process of plucking your eyebrows. Not only is it way too close to your eyes, but unless you have a hand steady enough for micro-surgery, you are going to suffer from accuracy problems smearing it on.

3. There is no one on Earth—not even Farrah Fawcett or Melanie Griffith—who looks good in a shower cap, so don't fret unduly about it.

4. The people who make toilet tissue have gone way overboard putting the perforations after every single square. We do not need that much exactitude and it gives small children the incorrect impression that one square could be sufficient. Tissue "folders"

and "bunchers" represent two very different personality types and should not marry each other.

Chapter

5

Laughing Your Way
To Good Health—
Afterword

Well, that pretty much wraps up my thoughts on Weight Control, or lack of same, Exercise, Motherhood and Housework. I hope that you have enjoyed several hearty laughs throughout this book or if you are of Norwegian descent, a couple of tasteful chuckles.

Researchers tell us that small children laugh up to 400 times a day, but as we "grow up" we learn that such spontaneous hilarity is improper and immature. Eventually we stifle that playful child in us until the average adult laughs but 15 times a day.

You may not have guessed from reading this book, but I am subject to infrequent but painful bouts of depression. Sometimes I get so depressed I question whether I *am* worth L'Oreal. I'm not even sure I'm "right for Grapenuts"; I fear someone will come and confiscate my cereal. I can tell you from my own experience with these episodes that I keep a good supply of "laugh medicine" with me at all times, even when I am on the road. Bill Cosby, Erma Bombeck, and Dave Barry are particular favorites of mine and I heartily recommend that you invest in their books.

I do not know if this is an original idea or not, but my friend Karen Kaiser Clark, an excellent motivational speaker, says that "People would worry a lot less about what other people think of them if they realized how infrequently they do!"

Loosen up. Do not worry about what the person in the adjacent cubicle at work will "think" if you whip out this book or a *Far Side* cartoon book at regular intervals during the day to charge up your laugh batteries.

Bobby McFerrin has made a fortune and indeed become a one-man industry with records, tapes, mugs, T-shirts, bumper stickers all urging people "Don't worry; be happy." He has been criticized and ridiculed for the utter simplicity of the message (by people who are probably kicking themselves around the block for not thinking of it first), but he obviously has struck a very responsive chord in people.

We live in a world fraught with personal and global stress and problems. The newspapers barrage us daily with terrifying and depressing information about the ozone layer, the disappearance of the rain forests, pollution, crime, divorce, disease. I am not suggesting that these are not real and pressing concerns, but living a humorless, grim life will not bring us one iota closer to solving these problems.

There is a good reason that the flight attendants tell us "in the unlikely event that there is a need to use the oxygen mask, PUT IT ON YOURSELF FIRST and then attend to your dependents." If you try to put masks on two or three children first, you will pass out before you can finish the job and be of no use to anyone.

In the spirit of concern for a troubled world, take care of your own mental health first. Take frequent laugh breaks throughout the day. Learn to laugh at yourself. Cultivate a sense of fun and play which carries over into all aspects of your busy life.

Laugh and be well. If you have enjoyed this book, I invite you to write to me at 3050 Presidential Drive, Suite 111, Atlanta, GA 30340. If you have *not* enjoyed this book, kindly give it to someone you hate.

And look for my sequel: Laughing Your Way Through Marriage, due out as soon as we sell all of these.

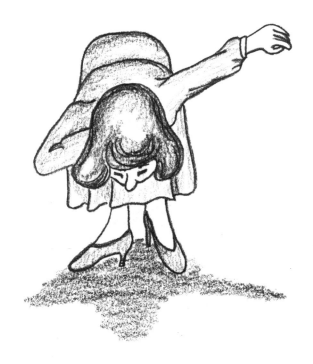